KU-794-292

THE
YOGA BIBLE

THE DEFINITIVE GUIDE TO YOGA POSTURES

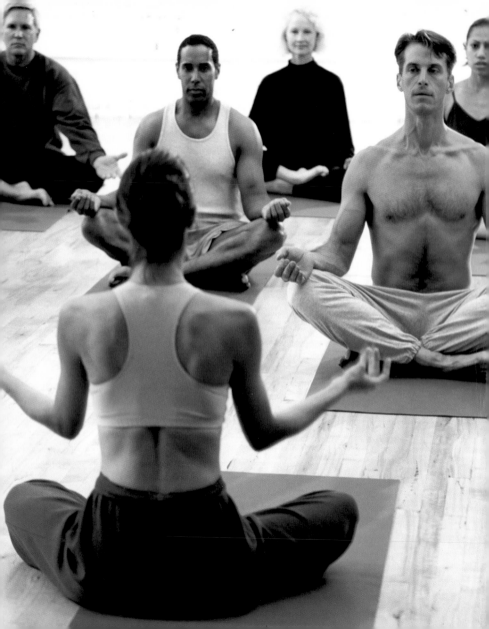

Part One

Introduction

Introduction

Yoga is learning to come back to yourself. It's finding your limits, expanding your boundaries, and being able to truly relax into who you are. It's about taking time to remember who you are but have forgotten while being caught up in the whirlwind of a fast-paced life. On a physical level, as in life, being off balance doesn't feel good. Feeling as though you might topple over at any time is neither safe nor comfortable. One of the reasons yoga has grown dramatically in popularity is that it helps you feel harmonious, integrated, and complete. As you learn about your center in a yoga pose, you practice finding your center in other areas of your life. In fact, dealing with a posture can train you to deal better with life events.

What is Yoga?

An author named Patanjali wrote *Yoga-sutra*, the first text on the subject of yoga, 2,500 years ago. In it he defined yoga as *chitta-vrtti-nirohdah*, which means the cessation of the turnings of the mind. The definition of yoga that I use most often is that of stilling the mind. It is the most common modern definition elaborated upon by the eminent teacher T.K.V. Desikachar, who stated that yoga aims "... to direct the mind exclusively toward an object and sustain that direction without any distractions."

Westerners and lay people usually think of yoga as its various physical postures. The name itself comes from the Sanskrit word *yuj*, which is often translated "to unite, to join, or to connect." All these associations imply reintegration and rebalancing, or bringing the self to a harmonious state. Other meanings of *yuj* include "to center one's thoughts, to concentrate on oneself, or to meditate deeply."

The practice of yoga helps us achieve inner stillness.

These tie in perfectly with the definition of yoga previously cited from the *Yoga-sutra*.

Yoga is actually a state of mind. Achieving the goal of stilling the mind is a tall order, so practices have been developed that allow you to move toward this state. Quieting the mind is a rather intangible goal. In contrast, the progress made on accomplishing a yoga posture can be evaluated by alignment, length of stretch, and the length of time it can be held. It's much easier for you to relate to something tangible— the body—and then move on to something intangible—the stillness of the mind. During yoga practice, you begin somewhere known and, using your body and breath, you move

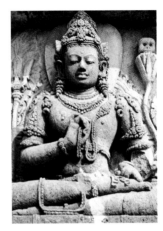

Buddhist meditation techniques can be applied during yoga practice.

toward an unknown. As you open your body and mind with yoga postures and breathing, you become receptive to the delightful and profound experience of inner stillness.

While the human mind tends to drift off into thoughts of the past or future, the human body exists only in the present moment. Hatha yoga, a type of yoga that emphasizes strenuous and persistent effort, encourages awareness of the body. Coming back to your body draws your mind back to the present. Then, worries drop away and there are no more "shoulds" or "musts." One of the reasons yoga is so refreshing is that, even if only for an instant, there is only the reality of the present moment. Each time you come to the present moment, you drop a certain amount of baggage. You may pick it up again shortly thereafter, but the point is that you have practiced letting it go. Eventually you will be able to reduce the stress more often and for longer periods of time. In this respect, yoga is like life training. Its practice is a fabulous tool for transformation.

The *Yoga-sutra* tells us that yoga consists of eight *limbs*—aspects of Hatha yoga (see page 380) practice that include codes of moral conduct, physical exercises, breathing practices, concentration (the ability to direct the mind toward an object and keep it there), and meditation (a state of one-pointed focus, see page 15). *Asana*, the use of physical postures, is the practice usually associated with yoga in the West. However, yoga may be anything that gives you a sense of unity, helps you better connect with yourself, and helps you remember who you are. It might be a walk along the beach, a luxurious yawn, or simply taking a single conscious breath.

Any practice that helps you center yourself is important. When you operate from a space that is close to your center, it is easier to be calmer and more focused. Being off balance is a huge source of stress. When things go wrong when you are already off balance, it is like swimming against a strong tide. The farther out you are, the harder it is to swim to shore. Yet, distractions and sensory stimulation often cause you to look outward rather than gazing inward. The real challenge in life is to manage to stay "with" yourself while at the same time interacting with others; to respond appropriately to people and events while maintaining a sense of connection to yourself.

The Rewards of Yoga

The continued practice of yoga brings medium and long-term rewards for the *bodymind*—the combined physical, psychological, and spiritual aspects of an individual. It also yields an instant feel-good effect. It just feels better to inhabit a looser, freer body than a contracted, tight, bound-up one. The human body was designed to move freely. By integrating all the parts that make up the whole self, practitioners often have a sense of standing taller and feeling freer. Afterward, they are relaxed and happily at ease. According to Indian philosophy, everything is a combination of three essential qualities called the *gunas*: *sattva* (a pure, balanced state), *rajas* (activity, restlessness), and *tamas* (inertia, laziness, depression).

The best yoga practice is when it is integrated into your life.

Most students start a yoga practice either in a restless or hyperactive state, or in a lazy or lethargic state. By the end of most practice sessions they have been brought toward an uplifted *sattvic* state, both mentally and physically.

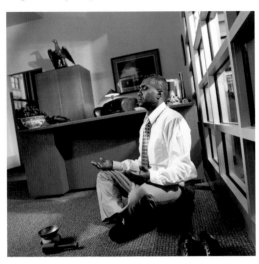

Yoga brings a sense of expansion on many levels. It allows you to rediscover an internal sense of wholeness that, in today's fast-paced world, is often lost. If you start with a restless body and a hyperactive mind that is difficult to focus, the appropriate practice will work out physical tensions and calm both mind and emotions. If you start with a dull, lethargic bodymind, the right practice will bring back a sense of aliveness to your body, refresh your mind, and give you a sense of peace. Every yoga practice represents a raising of consciousness that creates a reversal of its current state or condition. Whenever you truly come back to yourself, you have the chance to appreciate your essential wholeness.

Yoga gives you the tools to move from passion to the clarity of dispassion, from distress to de-stress, from dis-ease to ease. It unwinds you, moving you from a bound-up, contracted way of existing to a more easygoing, free-flowing way of interrelating. If your yoga practice expands you and gives you joy, then it is the right yoga practice for you.

The Eight Limbs of Yoga

The *Yoga-sutra* describes yoga as consisting of eight limbs. While the doorway into yoga for many these days is through the body by working with *asanas*, it is only one method. You may find yourself drawn to explore the remaining limbs as your practice progresses.

1. YAMA. The yama is a moral restraint that controls not only our actions, but also our speech and thoughts. As such, the yama is far-reaching and requires vigilance on the part of the *yogi* (one who practices yoga). Five are listed in the *Yoga-sutra*:

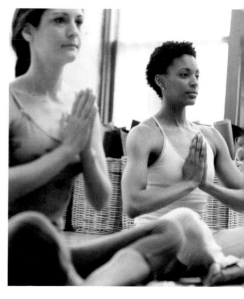

● **Ahimsa.** This term is often translated as "non-violence" or "non-injury." It includes compassion or consideration for all living beings. This precept includes your treatment of your body during your yoga practice. Overworking your body is neglecting to take care and, as such, is a form of misuse. Coax and persuade, but don't force your postures.

● **Satya.** This term deals with truthfulness. It includes the concept of appropriate communication—conducting your life with honesty in behavior, with thought, and with intention. It is important to assess accurately where you are at on a particular day before doing a difficult pose so that you do not push beyond your physical limit. Behaving in accordance with beliefs might mean that an environmentalist would not take a job with a multinational oil conglomerate or that a vegetarian would not work for a fast-food or burger outlet.

- **Asteya.** Often referred to as "non-stealing," asteya encompasses any avoidance of covetousness. This includes cultivating a less materialistic view of life and reining in desires for things that are not ours to have. Asteya includes not intimidating someone into doing or giving you something against their wishes or making copies of songs that would deprive artists of their royalties.

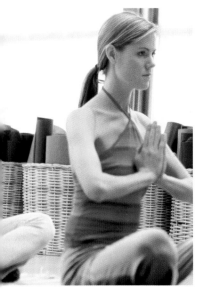

Yoga practice can be more wide ranging than just the practice of physical postures.

- **Brahmacharya.** Many take this concept to mean celibacy. Many spiritual traditions embrace celibacy as a tool for diverting energies away from sexuality and toward spiritual growth. Brahmacharya can also be interpreted as moderation of our actions and our search to fulfill our sensual cravings. It means avoiding the indulgence of the senses, choosing your sexual partners with care, and ensuring that your sexuality comes from a basis of love rather than inappropriate flirtation or manipulation. On a deeper level, it encompasses a commitment to, and a merging with, the Divine.

- **Aparigraha.** This might be defined as "non-greediness," since it encourages you to separate your true needs from what are merely desires or wants. Grasping life and material possessions makes lasting happiness harder to attain because the list of what you desire tends to spiral onward and upward. It is better to measure your success by who you are rather than what possessions you own. Instead of longing for more, it's also important to take time to appreciate what you already have: fresh air, good memories, healthy food, friends, a healthy body, or some uplifting literature.

2. NIYAMA. This means "rule" or "law." The niyama incorporates discipline in actions and conduct and in our attitude toward ourselves. Patanjali lists five:

● **Saucha**. This term means "purity" or "cleanliness." Aside from physical cleanliness and the cleanliness of your surroundings, it encompasses your diet and purity in thinking.

● **Santosha**. This precept of contentment offers us the opportunity to practice being satisfied with and appreciating what we have. It also encourages us to adopt a cheerful approach about things we don't have. However, while you may benefit from "looking on the bright side" and adopting an uncomplaining attitude toward an undesirable condition, don't use this precept as an excuse for accepting this state simply because you don't want to put in the effort to change it.

● **Tapas**. Originating from verbs meaning "to burn" or "to cook," this precept encourages you to develop a strong resolve and a burning enthusiasm both for your practice and for your life's work. Like the other precepts, *tapas* demands discipline, self-control, and persistence.

● **Swadhyaya**. This precept of self-study leads to self-discovery. *Swadhyaya* encompasses mindful self-reflection and continued outer learning through formal and informal studies.

● **Ishvarapranidhana**. Under this precept, you accept that an all-knowing principle exists. It reminds you that this higher force is all around you as well as within you, and this knowledge brings meaning to your life. In the yoga texts, no one god is named— that is left up to you. Some choose to honor an ideal rather than a single god.

3. ASANAS. The physical postures of Hatha yoga are what is commonly considered to be yoga in the West. In the *Yoga-sutra*s, however, Patanjali gives just three mentions of *asana*. The aim of *asana* is to purify the body and prepare it for the long hours of meditation necessary to reach *samadhi*. In this trancelike bliss state, the mind is able to remain focused on its object without distractions. By being one with the object of meditation, the practitioner experiences unutterable joy and peace.

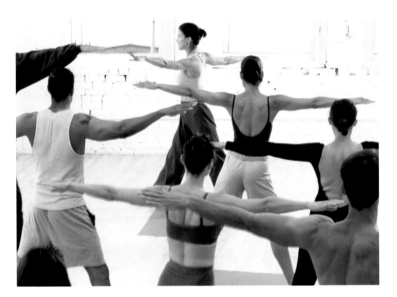

4. PRANAYAMA. This is the control of the breath aimed at cultivating the vital force (*prana*) within. (See the section on *Pranayama* pages 314–329.)

5. PRATYAHARA. This is the withdrawal of the senses. When the mind gains control over the senses, distractions from outside lessen and the mind can turn inward and focus on the other limbs of yoga.

6. DHARANA. This means concentration of the mind—the ability to direct the mind toward an object and keep it there. *Dharana* paves the way to the seventh and eighth limbs, *Dhyana* and *Samadhi*.

7. DHYANA. This is meditation, where the mind has a one-pointed focus.

8. SAMADHI. This is an illuminated state of absorption with the absolute. In this trancelike state, the turnings of thought are neutralized, the *yogi* gains control over the mind, and the thoughts are stilled.

Through working with the body, yoga teaches us to gain better control over the mind.

The Asanas

Yoga *asanas* are postures that rebalance the body. They bring strength to the weak areas of the body; they bring softness to the tight spots. They give you a workout, with the added bonus of a work-in. Not only do they create space in the physical body, they offer a sense of psychic spaciousness. By freeing up the outer body—the physical body, the muscles, bones, tendons, ligaments, and visceral organs—*asanas* build and control the *prana*, or vital force, of the body's subtle energies—energies that are finer and more subtle than those of the gross physical body that we can see. *Asanas* are considered to purify and heal the body as well as those subtle energies. Hatha yoga is great do-it-yourself preventive medicine.

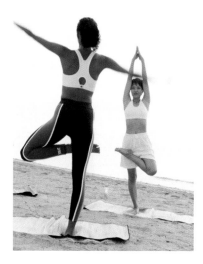

Yoga will increase your flexibility whatever your age or level of fitness.

The first thing people say to me when they discover I teach yoga is, "I'm not flexible enough for yoga." I often tell them, "That's why the rest of us do it!" Don't let a stiff body be an excuse never to start yoga. You should just start practicing from wherever you are right now. Don't judge your practice by how far you can or can't stretch. Never feel inadequate because you can't hold a pose for long, or because it doesn't perfectly mirror the pose in a picture. Practice spreading your awareness through your whole body. More than poise in your posture, seek grace in your breathing. Just start the journey. You never know where it might take you.

I use the term "edge" to describe the point at which the strong challenge comes into a pose and where you feel you have reached a new frontier. It's the point between comfort and discomfort, when you feel you have reached your limit. You will find that this point varies from day to day. You may notice your physical edge is different from your mental edge. Be flexible and adjust your practice to honor both. Move slowly as you approach your edge. As you hover there, your body will eventually release and open and present you with a new edge. Wait for your inner cue. Don't rush like a bull at a gate—that would be disrespectful. Be patient, and wait for your body to let you in.

Stay mentally present while you practice. Let your mind become absorbed in your work and in the subtle sensations of your body. Allow your practice to become a sort of conversation with your body. Be reflective, be respectful, be responsive.

Don't judge your practice only by how far you can stretch.

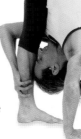

How to Practice

The instructions given in this book are those for the full version of each posture, but keep in mind that there is no "perfect" pose. Each individual can find his or her own health-enhancing way of performing a posture. Each special *bodymind* has its own special needs, and these needs vary from day to day, and even from minute to minute. Don't be disheartened if you can't perfectly replicate the photographed poses. Generally, throughout this book, the full (and most difficult) variation of each posture is shown. The pictures show some postures on the left and others on the right side. All asymmetrical poses should be carried out on each side of the body. You can choose which side to start. For many of the poses an Information Box is provided. This gives details about the pose under the following headings:

- **GAZE** The focus point for the eyes once in the pose.
- **BUILD-UP POSES** Preparatory exercises to help you achieve the full pose.
- **COUNTER POSES** Other poses that balance the effects of the pose.
- **LIGHTEN** Ways of practicing that make the pose more manageable.
- **EFFECT** The overall feeling of the pose.

Breathing

More than how deep you go in the postures, the essence of yoga lies in the breath. If you can breathe, you can do yoga. Get to know your breathing intimately. Better even than your best friend, know that your breath will always be there for you as you move through life. Good breathing is reassuring, soothing, and healing. It will bring your postures alive. Reconnecting with your natural breath will bring feelings of cleansing, lightness, and clarity. Holding the breath dulls awareness, creates tension, and impedes the feeling of flowing freedom that yoga brings to the bodymind. Conscious breathing within each posture keeps the mind alert and lets your practice be exploratory rather than routine. Conscious breathing with each posture will draw your mind to the present moment. Distractions are minimized once the mind is reined in and it becomes easier to find the essence of yoga—mastery of the mind and reconnection with yourself.

As your breathing becomes more conscious, you'll find it a useful tool to measure your proficiency in a posture. Once your breath stays steady, your *asana* practice moves closer to perfection. Let your breath be round and smooth during your *asana* practice. Should the breath cease to flow naturally and become jagged, jerky or forced, take it as a sign to ease off on the intensity of your practice. Incorporate Warming Breath (see page 332) into your posture work. A warming breath is one that stokes the internal fire and warms the system. The steady, pleasant sound of warming breath provides a point of focus for the mind and prevents it from dancing away.

If using Warming Breath becomes difficult, or if you feel it creates stress in the system, return to steady natural breathing. Should you notice that your breath freezes and you forget to breathe out, use circular breathing—a flowing sort of breathing where the breath is not held and there is no long pause between the inhalation and exhalation, or between the exhalation and inhalation. During my classes, I often remind people not to hold their breath in. Holding your breath is part of the natural startle reflex, and something that happens often as students find themselves in a new and strange yoga position.

Breathing through the mouth is rarely done during yoga practice. Breathing through the nose filters and warms the air before it enters the lungs. Let your breathing become intuitive but, in general, inhale when opening or unfolding the body, when you come up out of a pose, when raising the arms, or while twisting the upper back, or expanding the chest such as when bending backward. Most people find that exhalation comes naturally when moving downward, lowering the arms or legs, bending forward or sideways, or twisting the lower back.

Tenderly observe your breath and get to know your breathing intimately.

Throughout this book, the number of breaths is given as a guide to holding times for some postures. Because yoga is deeply personal, this is merely a suggestion. It's up to each individual to determine how long to hold a certain posture on a certain day.

How Often to Practice

Regularity is the key! It is better to practice a little and often than to practice for a long time rather irregularly. A natural starting point is once a week, but three sessions a week will bring more easily noticeable changes to the body. Should you embrace the philosophy, you might find that your yoga practice expands into your way of life.

For some people, yoga practice consists of a lot of negative talk about how they "can never do" a particular posture. That's not a great practice! Instead, spend time on build-up poses. A natural human tendency is to develop an aversion to the poses you can't do. Rather than running away from the poses that challenge you, choose suitable preparatory postures and work compassionately to extend your current limits. Practice doesn't always make "perfect," but it certainly does make you better at whatever you are practicing. And, just as with other areas of your life, if you don't practice something, you are less likely to get better at it.

Take heart. Yoga is not like Olympic-grade athletics or professional tennis. The wonderful thing about yoga is that you get better and better at it as you get older and older. People continue to improve physically (and mentally) for decades. Staying mentally aware and respecting your boundaries on the day-to-day level will prevent injuries. Finding your edge in a pose and waiting patiently to find your next edge will extend your limits. From there, your strength, flexibility, confidence, and focus will grow and grow. Remember, too, that yoga is a state of mind. Time will give you the benefit of wisdom as consistent practice increases your ability to quiet the mind.

The Intensity of the Practice

During your practice, intense sensations will arise. The sensations you get from a strong stretch are not necessarily bad, but do not force yourself into the postures. Discomfort is a feeling of working strongly that still feels positive. Pain is more acute than discomfort, and there is no pleasant element to the soreness of pain.

While discomfort produces a "good hurt," pain is a negative feeling and is counterproductive. Pain experienced while assuming a pose means that you have either overshot your limit by moving too quickly or that you are improperly aligned. Pain in the muscles or joints could lead to injury, so never ignore it. Come out of the pose and consult your teacher.

Remember that yoga seeks to bring you closer to your true, essential self. Rather than increasing pain, yoga aims to remove suffering. Pain and injury are signs that you have moved away from your pure, natural self. If your practice doesn't increase the joy in your life, it is the wrong practice for you.

How to Make Your Practice Easier

● Choose easier postures that are appropriate for your physical ability. The foundation poses are marked with the symbol ▲.

● Preparatory exercises are listed for each posture. Stay with the basic instructions and ignore the later instructions, which tend to increase the intensity.

● Keep your arms down rather than raised up in postures. Bend your knees when leaning forward, or when coming up from a forward bend to a standing position.

● Remember that regular practice is the key to success.

● Rest well between postures.

● Make your movements slow and breathe calmly.

Raising the arms and gazing up increases the difficulty of the pose.

A common response to a difficult physical position is to forget to breathe out. Rather than holding the breath in, establish a kind of circular breathing, or work with a steady, pleasurable, warming breath.

● Hold the postures for a shorter time. Rather than one long hold, try flowing in and out of a pose a few times. As you do this move in time to your breathing.

• Relax your muscles during the postures, rather than gripping them. In particular, keep your face relaxed, make sure your back teeth are unclenched, and adopt a soft gaze with your eyes.

How to Bring More Challenge to Your Practice

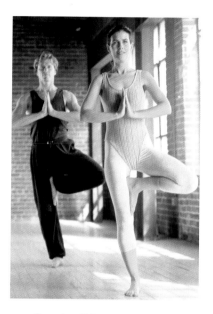

• Rather than working only the muscles necessary to hold you in a pose, work other muscles as well.

• Make an effort to firm, without over hardening, the muscles around the shoulders, knees, wrists, and ankles. Draw in the muscles of the lower abdomen to create Abdominal Lock (page 338). Incorporate Root

Engaging all the muscles in any pose will increase its degree of challenge.

Lock (page 340) and, where appropriate, Chin Lock (page 340).

• With awareness, follow all the written instructions that will increase the degree of difficulty in the pose. Sweep your mind over your entire body. From the tips of your toes to the crown of your head, aim to bring and hold your awareness of each part. Fully absorb your mind in your practice and the sensations of your body.

• Create a flow between postures, so you move from one posture to another in just one or two breaths. Use Warming Breath (page 332) for your entire practice session. Experiment with the more challenging postures but do not overstretch yourself or exceed your limitations.

Getting Ready to Practice

● Wear comfortable clothes and practice in a warm space. Having the feet bare brings more freedom to them. A sticky mat especially designed for yoga is a good investment. Rolling it out turns an ordinary room into your special practice area.

● Yoga is best practiced on an empty stomach. After a large meal, allow four hours before your practice. After a piece of fruit, allow at least an hour. Rather than taking fluids during the practice, hydrate yourself beforehand.

● When starting a yoga regime, decide how much time you are able to dedicate to your practice. Don't set yourself up for failure by choosing a routine that is not possible to maintain. Yoga, as a process of re-remembering who you are, works best if you do it little and often. The body responds best to a regular practice, even if that practice is short. You may well find that a fifteen-minute daily practice is more life-enhancing than a two-hour session once a week. Three sessions a week will really make you feel your body opening and coming alive.

● Never underestimate the "tiny yogas," the mini-yoga experiences you create in your day-to-day life. Try backbending over the back rest of your chair while seated at the office; create a steady Mountain Pose (page 46) at the bus stop; lengthen your exhalation in the middle of a traffic jam; do a single exhalation to soften the skin on your face when under stress; practice ankle rotations during a flight; close your eyes for a moment of quiet reflection between phone calls. Remember that "little and often" works best for the mind and soul. Continual reminders to reconnect with your self can never be underestimated. First, it becomes a habit; then it becomes a lifestyle; then it becomes who you are.

● Let your Hatha yoga session be a practice at being right where you are at that moment. Work in an uncluttered space and mentally close the door to distractions. While most people start with an idea of where they want their bodies to be, their practice has a tone of non-acceptance, since the body does not yet conform to their mental insistence that things need to be different from what they are. Your practice

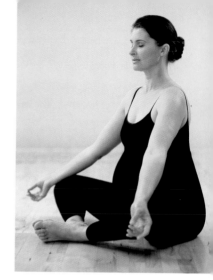

*Pregnant women can attend
specialized prenatal yoga classes.*

will be less enjoyable and harder to maintain
with such an attitude, which means you are less
likely ever to experience the true delights of
yoga. Don't practice for the future; practice for
the now. Instead of pushing with a "gritted
teeth" attitude, enjoy the yoga that is available
to you at this very moment. As a body-centered
practice, Hatha yoga is a sensual experience.
Enjoy it.

Structuring Your Practice

● Create a balanced routine by including an exercise from each of the following
categories: a flowing practice that develops your awareness of the breath; a standing
posture; a side stretch; a forward bend; a backbend; a twist; an abdominal
strengthener; a balance; an inversion; another forward bend; and always include
a final relaxation. *Pranayama* and meditation make a great end to a yoga session.
● If time is short, practice fewer poses with full awareness rather than hurrying
through many postures. Stay mentally receptive to the new things you can discover
in a pose. A childlike curiosity is a fabulous asset in life.

Special Conditions

● During menstruation, inverted postures, strong twists, and backbends should be
avoided. A gentle practice, including some supported forward bends and restorative
postures from the Yoga for De-stressing section of the book (page 354), are
beneficial during this time.

• While women find yoga a wonderful experience during pregnancy, it is best not to begin yoga during the first three months of pregnancy. For other health conditions, see the Yoga for Healing section (page 358) and, for assistance in developing a personalized practice, seek guidance from an experienced yoga teacher or yoga therapist.

Personal Perspectives on Yoga

I have been a yoga practitioner since 1989, and have written three previous books on yoga. I hold yoga teaching certificates from the Sivananda Vedanta Centre in India and the Sydney Yoga Centre. If you would like to find out more about me and my yoga classes, I invite you to visit the website of Yoga Source, the yoga center I founded, based in Sydney, Australia (www.yogasource.com.au).

I have seen many beneficial effects of yoga in my own life, some of which are intangible and difficult to measure, while others are more obvious. The most obvious benefit from my perspective is that the physical postures bring ease to aging or ailing bodies after moving, stretching, and limbering. As a qualified naturopath and counselor, I also have a strong interest in working with people to use yoga as a therapeutic method for those with respiratory problems, pain, nervous system disorders, or other physical limitations.

As you have already learned, yoga is far more than the ability to twist yourself into a position resembling an old mariner's knot. I believe that the physical postures also increase the flow of subtle energies. As you free up the body, you free up the mind. Flexibility in the body promotes mental flexibility, and this brings a sense of ease to life. In a similar way, a huge oak tree that stands stiff and straight will break in the wind and die, while a tiny sapling will bend to accommodate the wind and will thus live on. When you approach life from an easier state, you can more easily deal with the challenges it inevitably presents. I see and teach yoga very much as a metaphor for life.

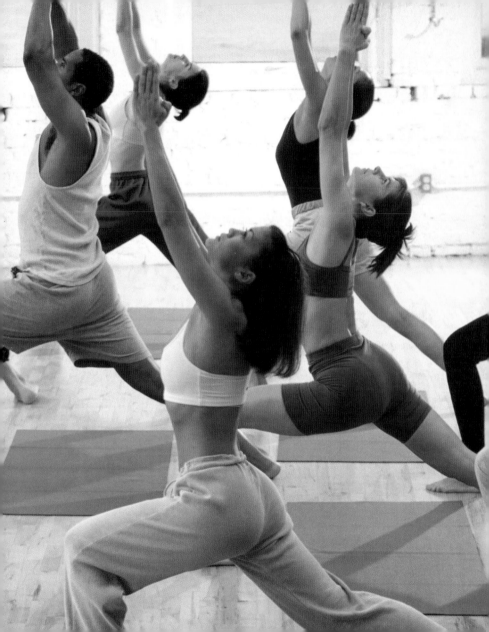

Part Two

The
Practice

Introduction

Yoga practice will develop awareness of your body's habitual holding patterns. Over time you'll start to find ways to undo less-than-perfect posture. With a balanced practice, your weak areas will grow stronger, and your tight areas will become more flexible. General vitality and energy levels will improve, and, as you unwind your *bodymind*, you'll drop into relaxation more easily. Yoga develops coordination, flexibility, stamina, balance, mental clarity, increased concentration and overall health. Yoga is an all-round life-enhancer.

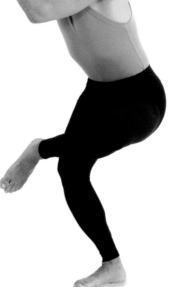

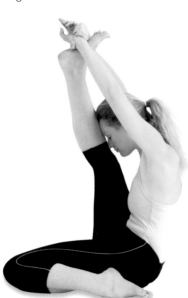

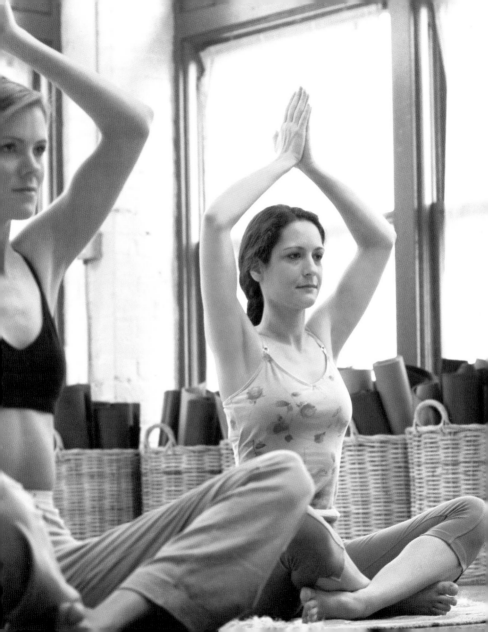

Preliminary Practices

While our bodies were designed to move, many of us lead such sedentary lives that we are missing out on the sort of limbering that comes from being physically active. It helps to warm up the body at the start of your yoga session to prepare it for the longer holding postures. As you warm up, you begin to put your mind into parts of your body that you may not generally think about much.

As you take a joint through its

range of movement, it works

the tendons and ligaments around it.

The circulation of fluids around and inside the joint

is increased. Increased oxygen, nutrients, and *prana*

benefit the health of the whole area and protect the

joint and cartilage from deterioration. On a purely

energetic level, these exercises unblock you by working

out any temporary interruptions to the flow of *prana*

around the body.

Cat Pose

Viralasana This pose may seem fairly easy. However, it develops concentration and awareness because you mentally visit the spaces between each of the vertebral joints to mobilize them. It also helps establish a steady breathing rhythm because you match the movements of the body to follow your breathing.

1 From an all-fours position, inhale as you lift your tailbone and head and make your back concave. Due to its structure, your lower back will dip down easily, but your upper back will become concave less easily. Rather than take the path of least resistance, stay mentally present and move the downward curve to the thoracic area. While all the muscles along the spine will be working, feel the muscles in the middle and upper back in particular switch on as you move your

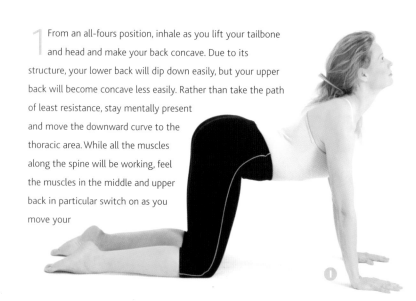

breastbone forward. Don't collapse into the shoulders, and keep the elbows as straight as possible. As you turn your face up to the sky, keep the back of the neck soft—if you had an egg cradled there, it wouldn't be squashed.

2 On each exhalation, round up your back. Let your shoulder blades spread wide apart as you release tight muscles of the upper back and neck. It is very easy to arch up the upper back, since that is its natural shape. During this part of the exercise, take care to press the vertebrae

of your lower back up to the sky. Tuck your tailbone well under and press your chin in to the throat. Press your hands to the floor and feel where the skin on your back stretches as you deepen your curve.

3 Move with a steady flow so that each rounding up takes an entire exhalation and each arching downward takes an entire inhalation. Once you get the feel for it, time the arching of your back so that the movement starts as you begin to inhale or exhale and ends just as your breath tapers out.

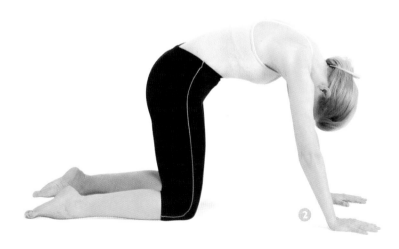

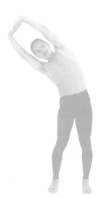

Sun Sequence

Suryasana After Cat Pose (page 32), which mobilizes the vertebral joints in the forward and backward direction, these two practices move the joints from side to side and in a twisting motion. As the name implies, they are a nice limbering practice first thing in the morning as you greet the sun.

1 Place your feet a little wider than hip distance apart and have your toes pointing straight forward. Inhale and bring your arms overhead, palms facing each other. Stay for a few breaths, letting the spine elongate. Tuck your tailbone under and draw your lower abdomen in toward the spine. Work into the shoulders by moving your arms back on each inhalation, then floating them back to vertical on each exhalation. As you consciously soften the shoulders, with each inhalation lift your heart center (located at your chest).

2 Interlace the fingers and press the palms away. On an inhalation, side bend to the right. Press the heel of the left hand away as you press against the floor with the right foot. Make yourself curve inward a little more at the right side waist and actively puff out your left side ribs. Don't let your upper arm move forward, but keep your body aligned on a plane. Get the sense of each vertebral joint side bending to its fullest. Inhale and come back to center, then exhale to the left. Consciously choose either to keep your hips centered over your feet, or to let them move in the opposite direction to your bend. Continue exhaling down and inhaling up for several rounds. On the last round, keep the legs very strong and hold each side bend for a few breaths.

3 From the center, exhale and twist to the right to look behind you. Stretch the heel of the left palm away. Have both hips even and level—press your right hip forward to increase the intensity at the trunk. Be aware not to collapse the left leg in, but hold it steady. If you like, tuck your tailbone under and feel how this changes the stretch in the lower back. Inhale back to neutral, then exhale to side two. Move between the sides five or ten times before holding for longer on each side. Maintain a firmness in the legs and intensify the twist from the base of the spine upward.

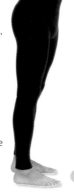

Neck Releases

The neck is a common storage spot for our tension. Apart from easing out stresses and strains, these neck-limbering exercises are useful after practicing Headstand (page 296), Shoulderstand (page 286), Plough Pose (page 292), and their variations.

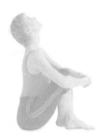

1 Sit erect and drop your left ear to the left shoulder. It is hard to let yourself let go of the head, so, as you stay here, remind yourself to let it be heavy so that the right side of the neck will lengthen. After thirty seconds or so, reach the right fingertips away to the side. Experiment with the position of your head and arm to get that "ahh—just right" feeling. It might feel better for you to move your right hand forward a little. It could suit you more to angle your face more toward the floor. Keep the sense of the head hanging. After some time, let your head drop forward to center. Let it hang a little. Rather than lifting the chin to lift the head up, inhale and move the back of your head up and back. Repeat on the opposite side.

2 Sit hugging your knees. First press the chin into the throat and lift the back of the head upward. 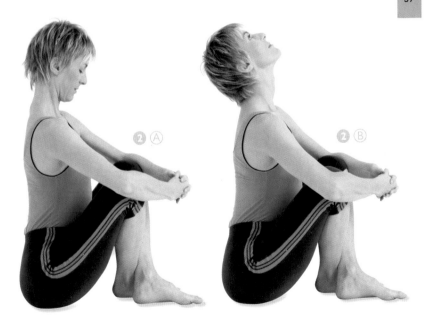 Ⓐ Move your shoulders down as well and you will feel the skin on the back of the neck stretch. Now concave the neck by stretching your chin forward beyond your forearms. Stay mentally present—consciously make the neck curve in as much as possible—it's rather like practicing a Cat Pose (page 32) using only your neck, rather than your back. Return to the first stage, tucking the chin in and back while visualizing the neck forming a convex shape. Ⓑ This neck release can be practiced in Downward Facing Dog pose (page 162), on all fours, and in Standing or Seated Forward Bends (pages 66, 74, 108, 122, 144, 146).

②Ⓐ   ②Ⓑ

Wrist and Forearm Releases

Wrists are often a weak point when trying to hold the Downward Facing Dog Pose (page 162) and the arm balances. Use these exercises as counter poses (poses that counteract the stretch of a pose) to relieve the strain created from a weight on the arms or long hours at a keyboard.

1 Kneel on all fours and place your hands so the inner wrists face away and your fingers point toward your knees. While keeping the palms pressed down, lean back to take the stretch to the inner forearms.

Hold and breathe. Release, and flip the hands so the backs of your hands are on the floor, fingers still pointing toward the knees. Lean back once again to stretch out the top side of the forearms. This stage is similar to Forearm Releasing Forward Fold (page 70).

2 From a seated or standing position, stretch your arms to the sides. Take your hands to Chin Mudra (page 334) by joining the tips of the thumbs and index fingers. Stretch

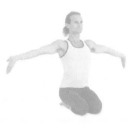

39

the other fingers
down toward the
ground. Then,
internally rotate
the shoulders,
turn your palms and
fingers to point backward, then upward.
(The inner crease of your elbows will be
facing down.) Now rotate the arms and
shoulders the other way so fingers point
forward, then upward. (Elbow creases will
face up.) You can either hold and breathe
at several stops or move slowly through
these positions to work your
entire range of
motion.

3 Start with your arms out to the sides,
palms facing up. Turn your fingers to
point down and toward your body,
as if you wanted to tickle your
side ribs. Press the heels of the
hands away. Unhunch your
shoulders and, to increase the intensity of
the stretch, move them forward.

4 Now rotate your palms so that
the fingers point up and
stretch toward your ears. Press the
heels of the hands away. While you hold
and breathe, drop your shoulders and roll
them forward and back to find a place
where it feels like you
get the best stretch.

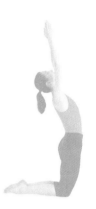

Sun Salutation A

Surya Namaskar A With practice, the movements become a graceful, smooth flow. Each movement is done on an inhalation or an exhalation using the Warming Breath (page 332).

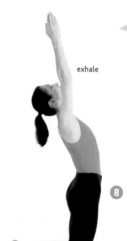

inhale

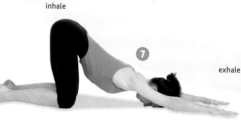

exhale

Kneeling Prayer Position
Re-centering yourself.
Become aware of your
breathing.

Kneeling Back Arch
Press the thighs forward
and lift up out of your
lower back.

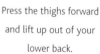

inhale

Extended Child Pose
Press back with the hands
to extend the hips away,
tailbone in the air.

exhale

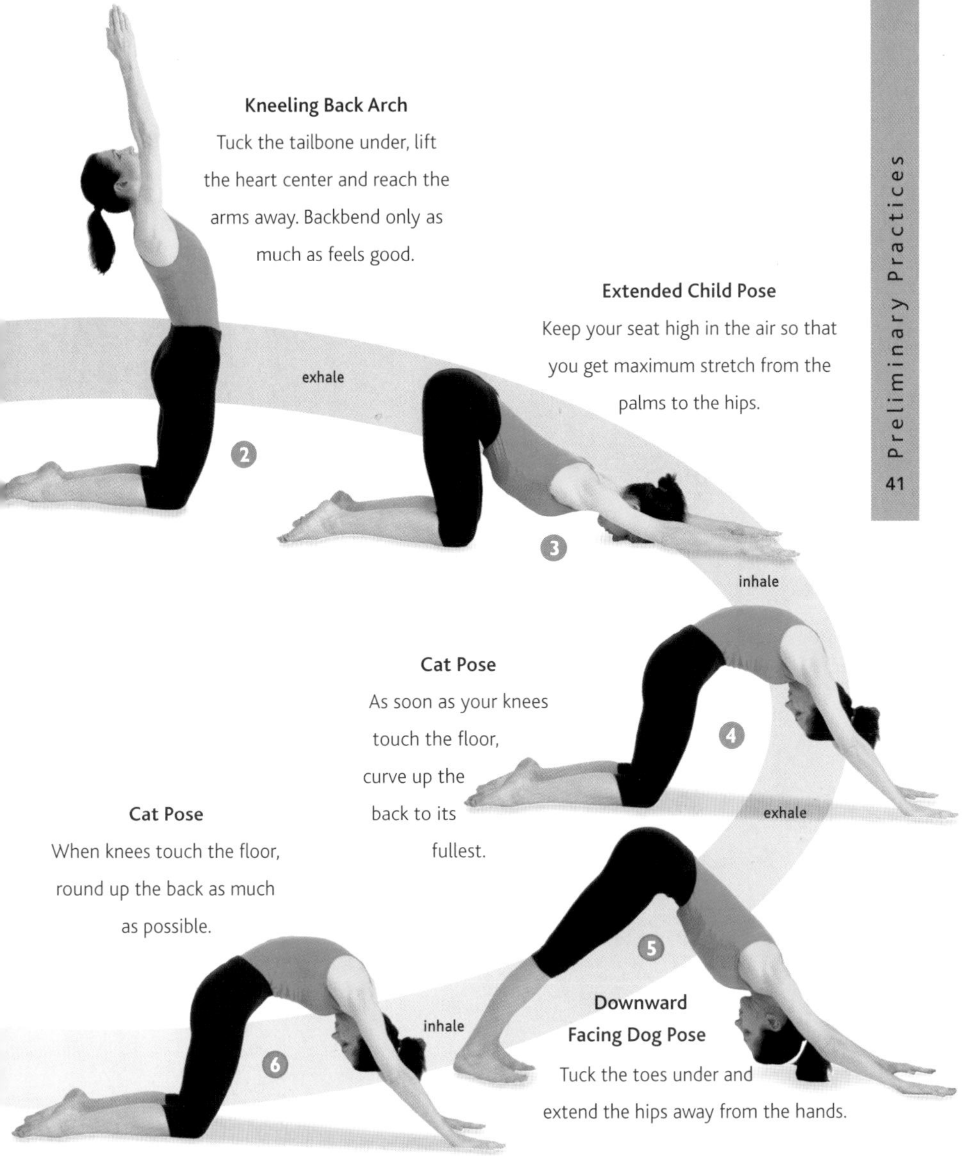

Kneeling Back Arch

Tuck the tailbone under, lift the heart center and reach the arms away. Backbend only as much as feels good.

2

exhale

Extended Child Pose

Keep your seat high in the air so that you get maximum stretch from the palms to the hips.

3

inhale

Cat Pose

As soon as your knees touch the floor, curve up the back to its fullest.

4

exhale

Cat Pose

When knees touch the floor, round up the back as much as possible.

5

Downward Facing Dog Pose

Tuck the toes under and extend the hips away from the hands.

6

inhale

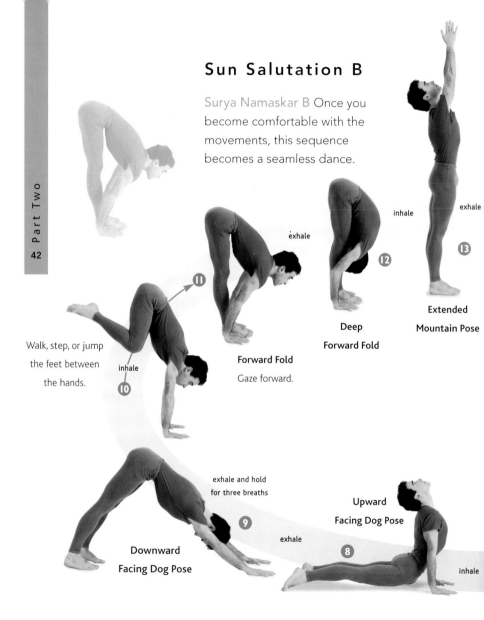

Sun Salutation B

Surya Namaskar B Once you become comfortable with the movements, this sequence becomes a seamless dance.

exhale

inhale

exhale

13

Extended Mountain Pose

12

Deep Forward Fold

11

exhale

Forward Fold
Gaze forward.

inhale

10

Walk, step, or jump the feet between the hands.

exhale and hold for three breaths

9

Downward Facing Dog Pose

exhale

Upward Facing Dog Pose

8

inhale

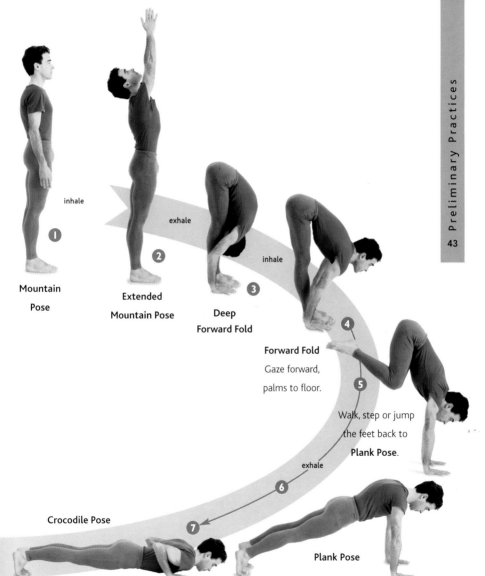

inhale

exhale

inhale

**Mountain
Pose**

**Extended
Mountain Pose**

**Deep
Forward Fold**

Forward Fold
Gaze forward,
palms to floor.

Walk, step or jump
the feet back to
Plank Pose.

exhale

Crocodile Pose

Plank Pose

Standing
Postures

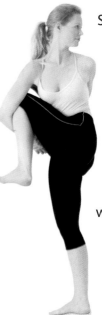

Standing poses have elements of
all the other poses; you can bend
forward, back, and to the side.
You can twist, balance, and even
go upside down. As stretched out
postures, they utilize large muscles,
warm the body at the start of
your practice and also develop
stamina. Standing postures demand
involvement from the whole body.

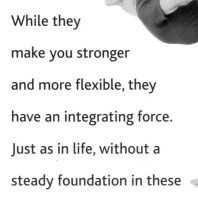

While they
make you stronger
and more flexible, they
have an integrating force.
Just as in life, without a
steady foundation in these
postures, you will never be able to extend to reach
your maximum. Standing poses teach you about
firm grounding, and only from there can you radiate
outward, blossoming to reach your full potential.

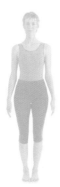

▲

Mountain Pose

Tadasana This pose is an invitation to stand tall with the majestic steadiness of a mountain. It is the basic standing pose, a place to start from and return to as we explore the more dynamic aspects of our practice.

1 Stand with the feet together. (A little farther apart is fine if you have lower back or knee stiffness.)

2 Close your eyes for a moment, and bring your mind into the soles of your feet. Rock forward gently over the toes and backward over the heels, coming to rest in a place where you feel absolutely balanced.

3 Spread the weight of your body evenly across your feet, heels to toes, and inner edge to outer edge. Make your contact with the floor as wide and full as possible.

4 Open your eyes, gazing forward to infinity.

5 Bend your knees slightly to awaken the legs. Straighten the legs slowly, bringing the knees directly over the ankles and the hips directly over the knees.

6 Bring your attention to the base of the spine.

7 Move the top of the front thighs back slightly, opening the area right at the top of the thighs where the legs join the trunk of the body. Draw the pubic bone in toward the core of the belly, so the bottom protrudes slightly. Then balance this movement by tucking the tailbone under slightly to bring the buttocks back into line.

8 Gently lift the chest away from the belly, feeling the spine extend upward through the crown of the head. Allow the shoulders to soften and drop away from the ears, and the very top of the chest to open. Let the arms be loose and relaxed beside the body, palms facing in toward the thighs.

9 Draw the chin slightly toward the throat, allowing the back of the neck to lengthen. Relax the throat.

10 Press down firmly through your feet into the floor and notice the equal and opposite flow of energy upward through the spine. Rest here a moment, residing in the vertical stillness of your being.

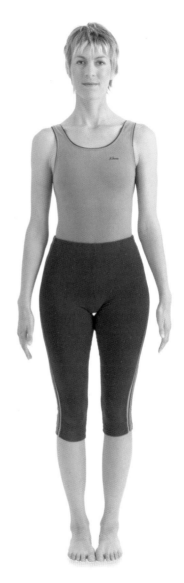

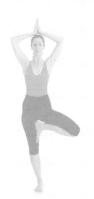

Tree Pose

Vrksasana As the roots of a tree provide the foundation for its body and branches, so our feet and legs provide the support for our upper body to stand with strength and grace. Balance poses demonstrate our state of mind. Focus is necessary to maintain a steady balance if the mind is jumping from one thought to another.

1 Stand in Mountain Pose (page 46) and draw your awareness to your feet. Gradually transfer the weight from your left foot onto the right foot. Visualize the sole of your right foot rooted to the earth.

2 Keeping the right leg strong and straight like the trunk of a tree, bend the left knee and place the sole of the foot against the upper inner thigh of the right leg, with the toes pointing toward the floor.

3 Bring your attention to the left knee and gently draw it back to open the left hip.

4 Lengthen your tailbone toward the floor and gently draw the pubic bone and lower abdomen toward the spine as you extend the spine upward.

5 Bring the palms together at the chest. If your balance is steady, inhale the arms up just above the crown of the head.

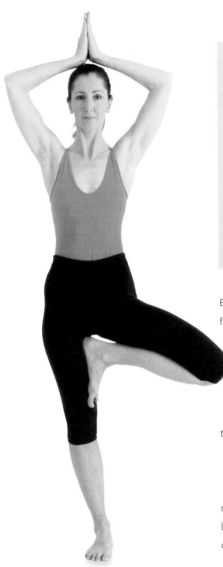

INFORMATION

GAZE Forward to infinity.

BUILD-UP POSES Mountain Pose.

COUNTER POSES Restful Deep Forward Fold.

LIGHTEN a) For easier balance, take the raised foot lower down on the supporting leg, possibly even with the big toe lightly touching the floor. **b)** Use a wall if necessary.

EFFECT Grounding.

Ease your bent elbows back, to open the front of the chest. At the same time, ease your bent knee backward to widen across the front of the pelvis.

6 Gaze steadily forward and breathe gently and evenly all the way down through the soles of the feet.

7 To release, lower the arms sideways to shoulder height and extend the right foot to the front, toes pointed as you lower the foot to the floor. Repeat on the other side.

Warrior Pose 2

Virabhadrasana II This pose honors
the heroic qualities that reside in each
of us. It connects us to the integral power
of our legs, which, linked with intent,
propels us to action. This is an excellent
pose to restore a feeling of power.
As you do the pose, silently say an inner
"Ha!" to your imaginary foe or problem.

1 Stand in Mountain
Pose (page 46).
Step the feet wide across the length of the
mat. Turn the left foot out 90° so that the
heel is opposite the arch of the right foot.
Turn the right foot slightly in—about 15°.

2 Square the hips to the front, tuck
the tailbone under and float the
chest and spine upward. Rather
than leaning your trunk to the
right, keep it facing forward, as
if you were standing in Mountain
Pose from the hips up.

3 Raise the arms to the
side. While you extend out
through the fingers, soften the
shoulders down. Turn the head to rest your

As you exhale, bend the left knee so that the left thigh is parallel to the floor. Make sure that the knee is directly above the ankle (not in front of it). Press the inner knee back so you can see your big toe, but not your little one.

gaze on the middle fingertip of the left hand. If your arms tire as they remain lifted beside you, focus on your inhalation. Imagine you are breathing through the fingertips and up the arms into the body or that you have balloons tied to your wrists, effortlessly lifting your arms up.

Build concentration by focusing on your front middle finger. Keep in mind that it's easy to forget what you can't see. So, at the same time, press strongly into the outer edge of the right foot, to keep the back leg strong and straight.

From the firm foundation of your legs and feet, lift against the force of Earth's gravity. Feel the strength of your own resistance, and then surrender.

To release, inhale as you straighten the right leg. Turn the left foot in and the right foot out and repeat on the other side.

INFORMATION

GAZE Tip of index finger.

BUILD-UP POSES Mountain Pose.

COUNTER POSES Restful Deep Forward Fold.

LIGHTEN a) Bend the front knee a little less. **b)** Keep your hands on your hips.

EFFECT Strengthening, focusing.

Standing Side Stretch

Parsvakonasana This pose engages the thigh muscles and awakens the inner leg from the groin right down to the ankles. Many of our day-to-day movements are simple forward and backward movements and we stretch sideways less often. Use lateral stretching to encourage lateral thinking.

1 Stand in Mountain Pose (page 46). Step the feet wide apart. Place both hands on the hips. Square the hips to the front.

2 Bend the right knee to 90° so the thighbone is parallel to the floor. Make sure the knee is directly above, not in front of, the hinge of the ankle.

3 Exhale and side bend the upper body to bring the right side ribs on top of the right thigh. Place the palm of the right hand on the floor beside the little toe.

Press the outer right knee against your right arm and rotate the abdomen and chest toward the sky. At the same time, press your right knee back against your arm to maintain maximum width across the front of the hips.

4 Reestablish your firm foundation by reinforcing the working of the legs. Press strongly into the outer edge of the left foot. Keep the right sitting bone moving back toward the left heel. Even while the right knee remains strongly bent, let the pelvis float (not sink) and take the minimum possible weight through on the right hand.

5 Extend the inner upper left arm over the left ear, palm facing the floor. Now push through the left side ribs so they curve up to the sky and awaken the stretch all the way along the left side of the body. Repeat on the other side.

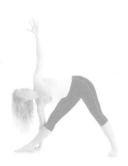

▲ Triangle Pose

Trikonasana This pose strengthens the legs and mobilizes the hips. It stretches the torso and opens the chest to allow for deeper breathing.

1 From Mountain Pose (page 46), step the feet wide apart. Square the hips to the front and lengthen the sacrum toward the floor, opening up the front of the hips.

2 Turn the right thigh, knee, and foot out 90°. Turn the back foot inward 15°. Raise the arms to shoulder height, palms facing down.

3 Inhale, extend upward through the crown of the head and out through the fingertips.

4 Exhale and extend the upper body to the right. Keep your right hip on the same plane as your shoulders and place the right hand as far down the front of the right leg as you can reach comfortably. Very flexible people may reach the palm behind the calf to the floor.

INFORMATION

GAZE Thumb of raised hand.

BUILD-UP POSES Mountain Pose, Gate Pose, Standing Side Stretch.

COUNTER POSES Downward Facing Dog Pose, Restful Deep Forward Fold.

LIGHTEN a) Keep the front leg bent, placing the lower hand on the thigh or knee. **b)** Place the back of the left hand on the sacrum at the base of the spine. Then focus on rolling the left shoulder back and opening the left hip upward as the buttocks tuck under. **c)** Look straight ahead or down to the floor if you experience neck discomfort.

EFFECT Enlivening.

5 Lift from the top edge of the right hip, lengthening the side ribs so that the spine and chest are helped to extend horizontally, creating the third side of the triangle.

6 Raise the left arm toward the ceiling with the palm facing forward and turn the face to the sky.

7 Revolve your navel upward. Open the chest, feeling a spiraling twist from the left hip upward through the spine, continuing out through the little finger of the left hand. While you breathe in this pose, extend and lengthen on the inhalation, increasing the twist on the exhalation.

8 The back of the body is one plane. Imagine the back of the head, shoulders, and buttocks are all pressing against a glass wall while you press your hips forward.

9 To release, inhale, allowing the upper body to lift you up to standing. Repeat on the other side.

Half Moon Pose

Ardha Chandrasana This standing
balance posture requires strength and
grace. Make use of your perfect mental
focus in this balance, and maintain it to
come out with control.

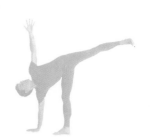

1 Start in a Triangle Pose (page 54) on the right
side. Take your left hand to your sacrum. Bend
the right knee and place the right fingertips on the floor,
about two hands forward of the right foot. At the
same time, slide the left foot toward the right heel, so
that your body weight begins to shift into the
right foot.

2 Breathe and stabilize your
foundation. Exhale and
straighten the right leg,
lifting the left leg up until
it is parallel with the
floor. Be stable and

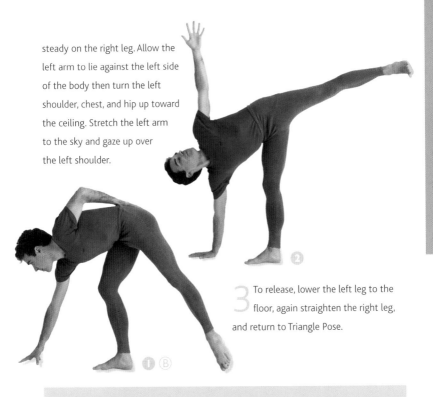

steady on the right leg. Allow the left arm to lie against the left side of the body then turn the left shoulder, chest, and hip up toward the ceiling. Stretch the left arm to the sky and gaze up over the left shoulder.

3 To release, lower the left leg to the floor, again straighten the right leg, and return to Triangle Pose.

INFORMATION

GAZE The top hand.

BUILD-UP POSES Triangle Pose, Tree Pose, Standing Splits.

COUNTER POSE Mountain Pose.

LIGHTEN a) Keep your gaze on the big toe of the right foot. Keep the left big toe lightly on the floor to develop your balance. **b)** Start with your heels positioned 4 inches (10 centimeters) from the wall and, in the pose, press with your buttocks and shoulders to the wall.

EFFECT Centering.

▲

Chair Pose

Utkatasana Squatting is an intensely powerful, innate body position that reminds us of our connection to the earth. Chair Pose works the muscles of the legs and arms and stimulates the heart and diaphragm. Strengthen your willpower by deciding in advance how many breaths you will hold in this pose—and keep to it.

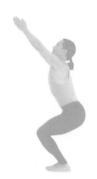

1 Stand in Mountain Pose (page 46) with the feet hip width apart. Inhale, extend the arms over the head and lengthen the spine.

2 Exhale and fold forward into Deep Forward Fold (page 68), bringing the chest toward the thighs and the hands to or near the floor. Inhale, bending the knees to bring the thighs parallel to the floor.

3 Press down into the soles of the feet and lift the arms and chest forward, away from the thighs. Keep lifting the chest, extending through the fingers until the arms, like the thighs, are parallel to the floor. Gaze straight ahead. Continue to breathe smoothly and evenly for four breaths. Lift the sitting bones up toward the ceiling (giving

your pelvis an anterior tilt) as you press down into the heels of the feet. You will feel the thighs working hard.

4 Exhale and bring the arms overhead and the spine to a more vertical position. Now tilt the pelvis the opposite way—tuck the tailbone under so it feels as if the lower back flattens out. Draw the lower abdominal area in toward the spine.

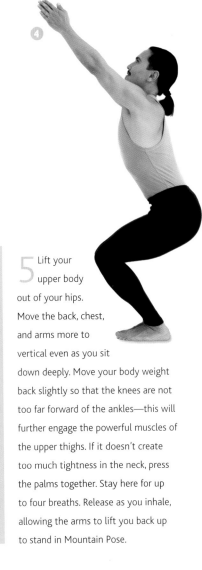

INFORMATION

GAZE Third eye or upward to infinity.

BUILD-UP POSES Garland Pose, Warrior Pose 1.

COUNTER POSES Deep Forward Fold, Restful Deep Forward Fold.

LIGHTEN a) Bend the knees less, especially if you have knee problems. **b)** Practice just the arm or leg action before combining them. **c)** Practice moving smoothly in and out of the pose before holding it for longer periods.

EFFECT Energizing.

5 Lift your upper body out of your hips. Move the back, chest, and arms more to vertical even as you sit down deeply. Move your body weight back slightly so that the knees are not too far forward of the ankles—this will further engage the powerful muscles of the upper thighs. If it doesn't create too much tightness in the neck, press the palms together. Stay here for up to four breaths. Release as you inhale, allowing the arms to lift you back up to stand in Mountain Pose.

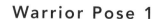

Warrior Pose 1

Virabhadrasana I This pose strengthens our connection with the grounding energy of the earth. This variation has an emphasis on establishing a firm and grounded foundation in the legs while fearlessly lifting and expanding the chest. As such, it is great for integrating the upper and lower halves of the body.

1 Stand in Mountain Pose (page 46). Inhale, step the feet wide apart, and bring your hands to your hips. Turn the whole right leg and foot out at 90° so that the heel intersects the inner arch of the left foot. Turn the left foot and leg in about 45°.

2 Turn the chest toward the right and square your hips by pressing your left hip well forward. On an inhalation, raise your arms above the head, bringing the palms together.

3 Exhale as you bend the left knee, sinking down into the right thigh and sitting bone. With your knee bent to 90°, it will be directly over the ankle hinge.

INFORMATION

GAZE Upward at thumbs.

BUILD-UP POSES Mountain Pose, Chair Pose, Warrior Pose 2.

COUNTER POSES Single Leg Forward Bend, Restful Deep Forward Fold, Mountain Pose.

LIGHTEN a) Look straight ahead.
b) Do not join the palms overhead.
c) Place the hands on the hips.
d) Bend the front knee less.
e) Have the front leg straight.
f) Lift the back heel.

EFFECT Strengthening, focusing.

4 It's easy to focus all your thoughts on what is visible in front of you. Spread your awareness to the back side of the body. From your front leg, take your weight equally into the back leg. Press into the left heel, feeling the stretch along the back of the right leg.

5 Let the tailbone drop down toward the floor to help in opening the front of the hips, the pelvic abdomen, and, front right thigh. This will also create space in the lumbar spine and help lengthen the lower back. Lift your head back and gaze upward. Once again, spread your mind to that which you can't see. Move from the back of the waist to develop your backbend as you stretch upward through the middle back and arms, even while you maintain your connection with the legs and feet.

6 Inhale as you straighten the left leg. Lower the arms as you step the right foot forward on the exhalation, returning to stand in Mountain Pose. Repeat on the other side.

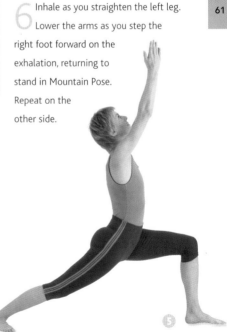

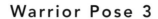

Warrior Pose 3

Virabhadrasana III This pose strengthens the legs and abdominal muscles. Just like all balance postures, it also helps to focus the mind. A fixed gaze will make you more stable. Create a mental line of energy that runs along the back side of the body. Use this to lengthen the heel of the raised leg to the fingertips.

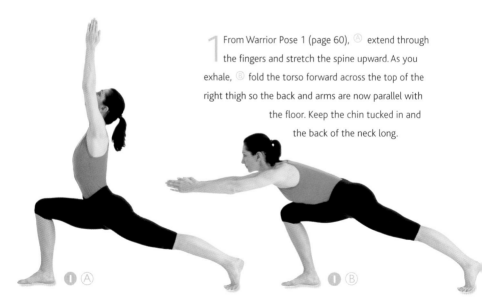

1 From Warrior Pose 1 (page 60), Ⓐ extend through the fingers and stretch the spine upward. As you exhale, Ⓑ fold the torso forward across the top of the right thigh so the back and arms are now parallel with the floor. Keep the chin tucked in and the back of the neck long.

❶ Ⓐ   ❶ Ⓑ

2 As you inhale, gradually lift the left foot off the floor until the leg is fully extended behind you. Rotate the outer edge of the left thigh downward, so both hips remain level with the floor and the sacrum fairly flat.

3 Straighten the right leg, pressing strongly into the big toe and spreading the sole of the foot wide across the floor. Stay here for five breaths, extending the energy of the spine forward through the fingertips and backward through the raised leg at the same time. Feel the strength and balanced beauty of this powerful pose.

INFORMATION

GAZE Beyond the hands.

BUILD-UP POSES Tree Pose, Half Moon Pose, Standing Half Bow Balance.

COUNTER POSES Deep Forward Fold, Mountain Pose.

LIGHTEN a) Do not do the leg lift, but keep the big toe of the back foot on the floor. **b)** Keep the arms extended backward, hands near hips. **c)** Use a wall to balance against.

EFFECT Focusing.

4 To release, exhale as you lower the raised leg to the floor. Inhale as your arms and chest lift up into Warrior Pose 1. Straighten the right leg and lower the arms as you exhale, stepping the left foot to stand in Mountain Pose (page 46). Repeat on the other side.

Revolved Half Moon Pose

Parivrtta Ardhachandrasana This standing balance pose strengthens the legs. The rotation of the torso provides a toning effect for the abdominal organs. From the abdominal center, bring the pose alive by sending lines of energy through each limb.

1 From a forward fold (page 68) bring the right hand to the floor in front of the left foot. With the left hand on the sacrum, bend your left knee and step the right foot back so your body weight begins to shift into the left leg. Breathe and stabilize your foundation through the sole of the left foot.

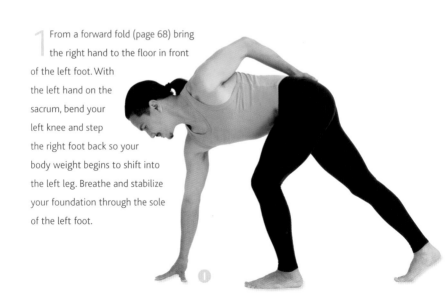

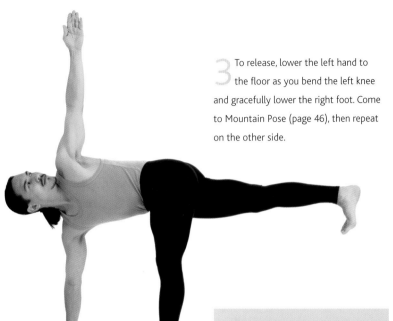

To release, lower the left hand to the floor as you bend the left knee and gracefully lower the right foot. Come to Mountain Pose (page 46), then repeat on the other side.

Look down to the floor as you raise the right leg off the floor and straighten the left leg. Using the right hand for balance, open the chest toward the left and extend the left arm upward. Extend the right toes down to the ground and stretch back through the right heel. Twist your trunk more to the left. If your balance is steady, turn the head up and gaze at the tip of the left thumb. Breathe deeply and evenly.

INFORMATION

GAZE Up to infinity.

BUILD-UP POSES Half Moon Pose, Revolved Triangle Pose, Warrior Pose 3.

COUNTER POSES Deep Forward Fold, Mountain Pose.

LIGHTEN a) Look down. **b)** Keep the back big toe on the floor. Bend the supporting leg. **c)** Practice parallel to a wall and press your hand against it.

EFFECT Balancing.

Wide Leg Forward Bend

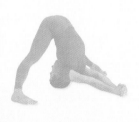

Prasarita Padottanasana In the urban landscape, the linear structures within which we live can inhibit the full expression of our range of movement. Spreading the legs as wide apart as they are able to stretch is immensely satisfying, and it expands the shape of who we are in the outer world.

1 Stand in Mountain Pose (page 46). Step the feet wide apart with the toes slightly turned in. Press the soles of the feet firmly into the floor so that both the inner and outer edges of the feet are fully engaged. Spread your weight evenly between the heel and ball of each foot. Allow the hands to rest on the hips. Inhale, tuck the tailbone under, and lengthen the spine upward through the crown of the head.

2 As you exhale, take your tailbone back and up to fold the upper body forward. Bring your hands to the floor, shoulder width apart, wrists in line with the inner arches of the feet. Allow the back of the neck to be long, and ease the crown of the head toward the floor as you let the weight of your head lengthen the spine.

3 Press into the outer edges of the feet as you lift the sitting bones up toward the ceiling, softening and lengthening the hamstring muscles at the back of the thighs. Bring your hips forward so the

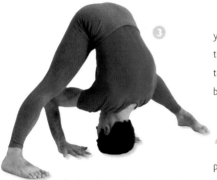

your shoulders, yet work the arms to bring the back of the head to the floor. If it does touch the floor, increase your challenge by bringing the feet closer together.

backs of your heels, backs of your knees, and sitting bones are in one line. Keep lengthening the front of the spine, lifting the ribcrests away from the belly on the inhalation as you fold forward more deeply with each exhalation. Unhunch

4 If you would like to include a shoulder stretch, from the upright position interlace the fingers together behind the back, if possible with the heels of the palms together. Lengthen the hands away from the shoulders, squeezing the shoulder blades together and rolling open the upper chest. Inhale and lengthen the spine. Exhale as you hinge at the hips and fold forward. Roll the shoulders away from the ears as you squeeze the shoulder blades together toward the spine and bring the fingers toward the floor.

INFORMATION

GAZE Tip of nose.

BUILD-UP POSES Deep Forward Fold, Single Leg Forward Bend, Wide Legged Easy Inversion, Bow Pose (for the arms).

COUNTER POSES Chair Pose, Standing Half Bow Balance, Camel Posture.

LIGHTEN a) Bend the knees
b) Place the feet closer together.

EFFECT Expansive.

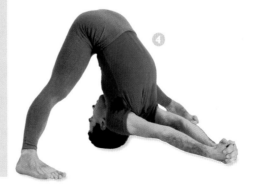

Deep Forward Fold

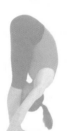

Uttanasana Folding forward from the hips gives the hamstrings and lumbar spine an intense, intentional stretch. Hanging upside down even for a few moments brings fresh blood to the brain and gives a refreshed sense of well-being.

1 Stand in Mountain Pose (page 46). Inhale as you open your arms wide, bringing the palms together above your head.

INFORMATION

GAZE Eyes closed or gaze softly at knees.

BUILD-UP POSES Head Beyond the Knee Pose, Double Leg Forward Stretch.

COUNTER POSES Locust Pose, Cobra Pose.

LIGHTEN a) To practice (Restful) Deep Forward Fold, take the feet hip width apart, bend your knees to rest your chest on the thighs and let your arms dangle.

EFFECT Re-centering.

2 Hinge at the hips to fold forward with arms lengthening forward and away from the tailbone. If your back is strong, keep the legs straight as you fold forward. Bring the hands to the floor beside your feet. If you can't reach, have the knees slightly bent, allowing them to gently lengthen with each breath.

3 If you touch the floor easily, walk your hands back and press more of your palms to the floor. Allow the back of your neck to be long, chin tucked in slightly toward the throat. Remain here for several long breaths, visualizing the spine as a waterfall, cascading forward over the rim of the pelvis as gravity lets the crown of your head gently move toward the earth.

4 Firm the lower abdomen and move the hips forward to inhale upward. Maintain the length in the spine as you lift the trunk upright to standing.

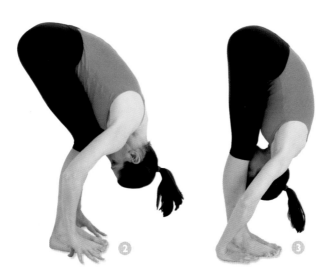

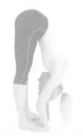

Forearm Releasing Forward Fold

Padahastasana This pose stretches the front of the forearms and provides an excellent counter pose to any posture where the palms take weight. Since the spine is stretched forward to its maximum length, the hamstrings receive a great stretch.

1 Stand in Mountain Pose (page 46). Bring hands onto hips, inhale and lengthen the spine upward.

2 Exhale and, keeping the length in the spine, turn the tail up and fold forward from the hips, bringing the fingertips to the floor near the feet. Spend several breaths here warming up into the hamstring stretch.

3 Inhale, raise the head, and look forward as you lift the chest away from the thighs. Keep your fingertips touching the floor and use them like anchors as you pull your side ribs through your upper arms and flatten the back. Press the sitting bones backward and lengthen the spine forward toward the crown of the head at the same time.

4 Bend your knees, lift the balls of the feet off the floor, and one by one tuck your hands under your feet, fingers toward the heels, inner wrists in line with the top of the toes.

5 On the exhalation, once again fold the upper body deeply toward the thighs, bringing the forehead toward the knees. Bend your elbows toward your shinbones or just past them to maximize the forearm release. Draw the shoulder blades down the back, pressing the shoulders away from the ears and freeing the neck. Move the sitting bones upward as you press down more with the toes. Distribute your weight evenly between your left and right foot.

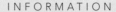

INFORMATION

GAZE Tip of nose.

BUILD-UP POSES Deep Forward Fold, any forward bend.

COUNTER POSES Mountain Pose, Standing Half Bow Balance, any palm balancing posture.

LIGHTEN a) Bend the knees.
b) Stand with a wall behind you. Have your heels one foot from the wall and lean your buttocks against the wall.

EFFECT Calming.

6 On the inhalation, activate Abdominal Lock (page 338) by gently squeezing the pubic abdomen in toward the spine. On the exhalation move your floating ribs farther down the thighs toward your knees and press open the back of the legs.

7 Bring your hands onto your hips, firm the lower abdominal area as you move your hips forward to stand up, and come back to Mountain Pose.

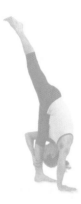

Standing Splits

Urdhva Prasarita Eka Padasana
This pose stretches the back of the
legs and improves the circulation in
the abdominal organs. As an inverted,
forward bending posture it requires
flexibility, focus, and a steady anchoring.

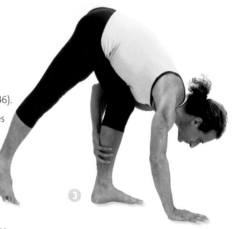

1 Stand in Mountain Pose (page 46).
Inhale and as you press the soles
of the feet firmly into the floor, feel
the spine lengthen upward from
the tip of the tailbone to the
crown of the head.

2 Exhale and fold forward from the
hips, keeping the length in the spine
and bringing the palms to the floor under
your shoulders, knees bent if necessary.

3 Slowly shift the weight of the body
into the left foot. Keep the right palm

or fingertips on the floor, and move your
left hand and forearm to the left calf,
elbow pointing back behind the knee. Press
your front ribs to your left thigh. Step the
right foot back slightly, keeping the big toe
on the floor for balance.

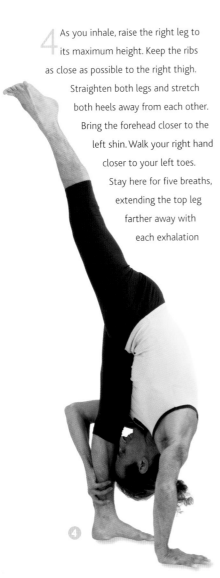

4 As you inhale, raise the right leg to its maximum height. Keep the ribs as close as possible to the right thigh. Straighten both legs and stretch both heels away from each other. Bring the forehead closer to the left shin. Walk your right hand closer to your left toes. Stay here for five breaths, extending the top leg farther away with each exhalation

INFORMATION

GAZE Tip of nose.

BUILD-UP POSES Deep Forward Fold (or any forward bend), Revolved Half Moon Pose, Raised Leg Downward Facing Dog Pose.

COUNTER POSES Mountain Pose, Standing Half Bow Balance.

LIGHTEN a) Keep the left big toe lightly touched to the floor behind you if your balance is unsteady.
b) Bend the supporting leg.
c) Keep both hands on the floor, well in front of your right foot.

EFFECT Centering.

5 Returning the right foot gracefully to the floor behind you, step the feet together and place both hands on the floor under the shoulders. From this folded forward position repeat on the other side.

Single Leg Forward Bend

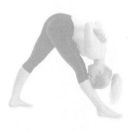

Parsvottanasana This standing forward bend is excellent for opening both the hip and shoulder joints. It provides a strong stretch for the back of the legs and gently contracts the abdominal organs.

1 In Mountain Pose (page 46), tuck the tailbone under and open the front of the hips. Gently draw the pubic abdomen in toward the spine. Lift the crests of the ribs away from the upper belly and allow the whole front of the body to lengthen and open. Soften the shoulders and allow the back of the neck to be long as the crown of the head lifts toward the ceiling.

2 Take your arms out to the sides and rotate the shoulders forward so the thumbs turn down.

3 Take the hands behind the back and bring the palms together (in prayer—namaste—position) to the middle back behind the heart. Press the outer edge of the hands into the spine as you pull the inner elbows back and roll open the front of the shoulders. Take a deep inhalation, enjoying the expansion available in the chest.

4 Step the left foot back. For easier balance, keep the feet hip width apart; otherwise, position the arch of the left foot in line with the left heel. Turn the left foot a little out to the side. Square the hips to face the front.

5 On an exhalation, hinge at the hips to fold forward. Keep the chin tucked in, back of the neck long, forehead toward the right knee. Bring the navel toward the right thigh and aim the forehead toward and beyond the right knee. Keep both legs strong and straight. Suck the right front thigh muscles in to the bone and press the outer edge of the left foot into the floor.

INFORMATION

GAZE Tip of nose.

BUILD-UP POSES Deep Forward Fold, Head Beyond The Knee Pose, Cow Posture (arms).

COUNTER POSES Mountain Pose, Standing Half Bow Balance, East Stretch Posture, Supported Bridge Pose.

LIGHTEN a) Place the hands on the hips. **b)** Hold your elbows behind the back. **c)** Bend the front knee. **d)** Fold forward only until your spine is parallel to floor, keeping your chin tucked in.

EFFECT Releasing.

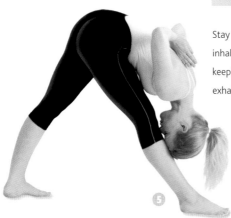

Stay here for several breaths. On each inhalation, lengthen the spine while keeping the hips square. On each exhalation, deepen into the forward fold.

6 Inhale to raise the upper body to standing. Step the left foot forward to stand in Mountain Pose. Repeat on the other side.

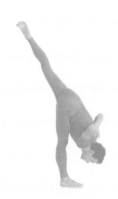

Single Leg Swan Balance

Eka Pada Hamsa Parsvottanasana This extended version of Single Leg Forward Bend adds to the complexity of the pose the challenge of balancing. Remember that balance is intrinsically connected to mental focus, so steady yourself to bring a swan-like grace to the posture.

1 Practice Single Leg Forward Bend (page 74). Once you have folded forward fully so your torso is over the front leg, squeeze the wings of the elbows toward each other, opening the front of the shoulders. Press the mound of the thumbs closer together. If your back is strong and you would like a more challenging version of this sequence, complete it with fingers interlaced behind the head as pictured. Hold for five breaths.

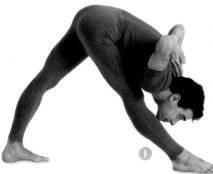

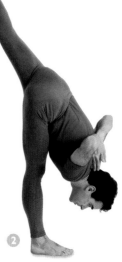

2 Once you have bent forward as far as you can go, transfer more weight onto your front foot and raise the back leg in the air. Let the back leg act like a stabilizing rudder. Earth down through the ground with the supporting leg, and press up to the sky with the other foot. Press both heels away from each other and let the

pose integrate well into the hips. Stay for five steady breaths.

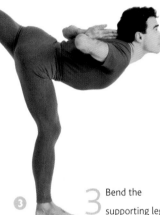

INFORMATION

GAZE To floor or ahead to infinity.

BUILD-UP POSES Single Leg Forward Bend, Deep Forward Fold, Head Beyond the Knee Pose, Standing Splits.

COUNTER POSES Stage 3 of the sequence, Mountain Pose, Standing Half Bow Balance.

LIGHTEN a) Gaze at a fixed point. **b)** Hold your elbows behind your back or stretch the arms straight back, fingers extending past hips. **c)** Keep your back foot on the floor. **d)** Hold for a shorter time.

EFFECT Focusing.

3 Bend the supporting leg and raise the torso so that your chest and shoulders are higher than your hips. Concave the back and keep your chest high so you activate the muscles along the spine. This pose is called Unsupported Swan Pose, and it acts as a counter pose to the back, after the Forward Bend. Remain here for five breaths.

4 Bring the raised foot to join the front foot as you raise your torso up to Mountain Pose (page 46). Repeat on the other side.

Revolved Triangle Pose

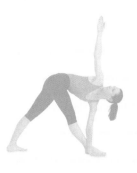

Parivrtta Trikonasana Fold forward and twist deeply in this standing posture. Use this posture to practice grounding through the feet as your foundation for a full extension. You will find that the farther you bend and twist, the more challenging the position becomes.

1 Stand in Mountain Pose (page 46). Step the feet wide apart and turn the right foot out so that the heel points toward the inner arch of the left foot. Turn the toes of the left foot well in toward the right foot. Square the hips to the front, tuck the tailbone under, and lengthen the spine toward the crown of the head. Inhale, raise the arms to shoulder height, and open the chest.

2 As you exhale, swing the chest toward the right leg and bring the palm of the left hand to the floor outside the right foot. Keep spiraling upward through the upper body as you twist the left ribs toward the right thigh. Lift the right hand toward the ceiling, extending through the fingertips, palm facing forward.

3 Turn the head and gaze upward in the direction of the right hand, keeping the back of the head in line with the spine and the length along the back of the neck. Press the right sitting bone backward and up, keeping the sacrum level. Press strongly into the outer edge of the back foot.

4 Lengthen the right side waist by moving the right hip and armpit away from each other. As you inhale, create space in the spine, extending back through the sitting bones and forward through the crown of the head at the same time. Feel the chest expand.

5 As you exhale, gently draw the abdominal muscles in toward the spine and spiral deeper into the skyward twist. Breathe here for five breaths. Inhale and untwist the same way as you came into the pose. Repeat on the other side.

INFORMATION

FOCUS Top hand.

COUNTER POSES Chair Pose, Mountain Pose.

BUILD-UP POSES Single Leg Forward Bend, Deep Forward Fold, Revolved Easy Pose.

LIGHTEN a) Bend the front knee.

b) Place the lower hand near the floor to the shin or the big toe side of the foot. **c)** Place the upper hand on the sacrum. **d)** Gaze at the floor or straight ahead, rather than up. **e)** Placing the feet closer together makes it easier to balance.

EFFECT Balancing.

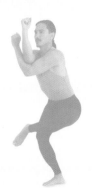

Eagle Pose

Garudasana This standing balance pose strengthens the ankles and is excellent for releasing tightness in the shoulders. Balance poses give a sense of poise and steadiness and are particularly beneficial when you feel mentally stressed.

1 Stand in Mountain Pose (page 46). Spend a few moments allowing the soles of the feet to connect evenly and fully with the floor. Deeply bend the right knee as you gradually transfer the weight of the body onto the right foot.

2 Lift the left leg, cross it over the right knee, then twist the front of the left foot around the right calf. Catching the foot around the calf will only be possible if your supporting leg is bent.

3 Sit down a little into the buttocks so that the right knee bends more deeply. Tuck the tailbone under and extend the spine upward, so that the upper body is lifting vertically. Tuck in the chin toward the throat, keeping the back of the neck long.

4 Inhale and extend the arms forward at shoulder height. Cross the right

arm over the left, then fold the forearms upright at the elbows and wrap them around to bring the palms of the hands together. Lift the elbows to shoulder height as you extend the hands away from the face. Relax the shoulders away from the ears, pulling the shoulder blades down the back.

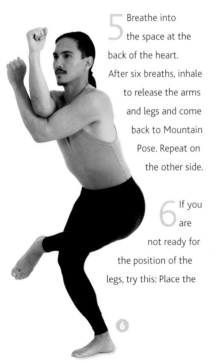

5 Breathe into the space at the back of the heart. After six breaths, inhale to release the arms and legs and come back to Mountain Pose. Repeat on the other side.

6 If you are not ready for the position of the legs, try this: Place the

INFORMATION

GAZE Hands.

BUILD-UP POSES Mountain Pose on tiptoes, Half Lotus Toe Balance, Revolved Triangle Pose, Downward Facing Dog Pose, Cow Posture.

COUNTER POSES Wide Leg Forward Bend with fingers interlaced, Cat Pose.

LIGHTEN a) Simply cross the left leg over the right and allow the toes of the left foot to rest against the outer right ankle if you cannot wrap foot around the back of the right leg. **b)** For balance, practice with the back against a wall. **c)** Practice the arm and leg positions separately.

EFFECT Focusing.

outer left ankle on the right thigh just above the knee. Let the knee move out to the side and bend the supporting leg more to a squat. If your palms don't come to press together, make two fists and move the back of the wrists to face each other, as pictured.

Revolved Side Angle Stretch

Parivrtta Parsvakonasana As a standing pose, this twisting posture is very grounding. The twist, which requires a high degree of flexibility, strongly squeezes the abdominal organs. The massaging helps digestive function and improves bowel elimination.

1 From a kneeling position, take your right leg forward to a lunge. Place the left hand on the outer right knee and the right hand on your hip. Stay here for several breaths, letting the spine lengthen upward. Next, begin to twist the hand against the knee, while resisting with the knee.

2 Draw in the lower abdomen once more as you lift the front of the torso and take your left hand to the floor by the right little toe. Your right knee will be close to the armpit. Rather than having your chest facing the floor, move it more to the side using the pressure of the left arm and right leg against each other. With your right hand on the sacrum, tuck your back toes under and lift your back knee off the floor. Extend well through the left heel as you move the back of your left knee skyward. Gaze beyond the right shoulder.

Once steady in the twist, turn the head to look past the armpit toward the sky.

4 Keep the back of the neck long and the back of the head in line with the spine. Rather than letting the left hip drop, raise it up a little.

3 Turn the left heel in and press it down. Press the outer edge of the foot against the floor. Sweep your right arm overhead, palm facing towards the floor.

5 Stay in the twist for a few breaths. On each inhalation, stretch more from the fingertips of the raised hand to the outer edge of the back foot. On each exhalation, draw the abdominal muscles toward the spine. Open the chest upward to deepen the twist. Inhale up out of the pose and repeat on the other side.

INFORMATION

GAZE Fingertips or straight up to sky.

BUILD-UP POSES Revolved Triangle Pose, Revolved Half Moon Pose, lunges.

COUNTER POSES Wide Leg Forward Bend, Downward Facing Dog Pose.

LIGHTEN a) Stay at first and second stage. **b)** Bring the left elbow (or armpit) to the outer edge of the right knee, palms together in prayer position, thumbs at the breastbone. **c)** Take the bottom hand to the big toe side of the front foot.

EFFECT Energizing.

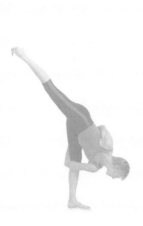

Side Angle Pose Sequence

Nirlamba Parsvakonasana This standing lateral stretch strengthens the thighs and expands the chest and lungs. It can also increase the range of movement available in the shoulders. It is a real dance between extension and stability—stretching to your maximum without toppling over.

1 Step the legs wide apart. Turn the left foot out 90° and turn the right foot in about 15°. Bend the left knee to a right angle. Stretch the arms out to the sides and lengthen through the sides of the trunk. Extend through the left side of the trunk, as you exhale and bring the left hand to the floor by the big toe so you are in Standing Side Stretch (page 52).

2 Have the back of the right hand resting at the base of the spine. Inhale and lengthen the left side ribs along the inner left thigh. Lift the chest and pull the right shoulder down and back to open the front of the body. Tuck the left buttock down and under, bringing the whole back of the body, from the right heel right up to the back of the head, more onto one plane.

3

3 Internally rotate the left shoulder as you bend the elbow, so the hand starts to move underneath the left leg. Take the hand up toward the lower back and grasp the right wrist with the left hand. On the exhalation, increase the rotation of the chest toward the ceiling. Press your left elbow against the knee and the knee back against the elbow. Accentuate this rotation further by pulling the right wrist back away from the left knee, as if trying to straighten both elbows. Turn the head to look up to the sky. Stay here for a few breaths and bring your focus to different parts of the stretch with each breath.

4 Now loosen your grasp a little to lock just the curled fingertips together. Look down to the floor. Step the back foot in and come to balance on the back big toe. If possible, lift the back leg in the air. Straighten it as you stretch your heel away as much as possible. Straighten your supporting leg. Stretch the soles of the feet away from each other. Stay for five breaths. Come back to Step 1, then inhale your torso up, to practice on the other side.

INFORMATION

GAZE First stage—skyward. Second stage—floor.

BUILD-UP POSES Warrior Pose 2, Standing Side Stretch, Half Moon Pose, Sage Twist 1.

COUNTER POSES Wide Leg Forward Bend, Resting Deep Forward Fold, Mountain Pose.

LIGHTEN a) Bring the left elbow just to the top of the left knee. **b)** Extend the right forearm behind the back and tuck the fingers above the left hip crease before bringing the left hand to floor. **c)** Keep back foot lightly on the floor to develop your balance.

EFFECT Focusing.

One Legged Garland Pose

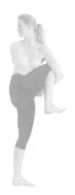

Eka Pada Malasana This challenging pose works the abdominal muscles, gives the organs a good workout and helps open the shoulders. As it is the standing and balancing version of the Seated Bound postures, it demands a more acute mental focus.

1 Stand in Mountain Pose (page 46). Transfer the weight of the body onto the left foot and bend the right knee up toward the chest. Find your balance and the initial stretch by hugging your knee to your chest.

2 Reach the right arm forward past the inner leg, bringing the underarm snug against the inside of the right knee. Internally rotate the arm from the shoulder and wrap the forearm around the outside of the right shin, bringing the back of the right hand beside the right hip to lock in the leg.

3 Lift the heart and lengthen the spine upward as you raise the left arm to the side and spiral the palm to face backward. On your next exhalation, twist the upper body to the left and extend the

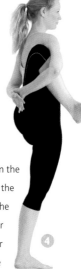

left arm behind the waist. Clasp the left wrist with the right hand.

4 Take five breaths here, facing forward and standing tall. Help the shoulders and the heart to open by working the hands away as if you wanted to straighten the elbows. Stretch the toes of the raised foot. Release with control.

5 For the twisted version, Revolved One Legged Garland Pose, once again hug the right knee in to the chest. Inhale, bring the left arm high up and, turning from the lower belly, twist the trunk deeply to the right. Bend the left elbow and bring the back of the left shoulder to the outer right knee. Rotate the left arm internally, so the elbow points up. Then wrap the knee with the arm as you bring the left hand near the left hip. Once the knee is wedged in, reach the right arm around it to clasp the right wrist with the left hand. Turn your head to look back. Increase the intensity by lifting yourself up to stand taller. Straighten the supporting leg well. Try to straighten the elbows. Stretch out all the toes of the right foot.

INFORMATION

GAZE First stage, straight ahead. Second stage, far to the side.

BUILD-UP POSES Seated Half Spinal Twist, Sage Forward Bend A, Sage Forward Bend C, Noose Posture.

COUNTER POSES Chair Pose, Restful Deep Forward Fold, Mountain Pose.

LIGHTEN a) Simply hug knee to chest **b)** Use a belt to link the hands. **c)** Practice it seated.

EFFECT Focusing.

Half Lotus Toe Balance

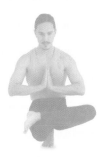

Padangustha Padma Utkatasana In this standing balance, the heart remains a focus as you sink down into the supporting leg and gently allow the hip of the bent leg to open with the breath. It helps strengthen the ankles and bring flexibility to the hips and develops balance and clarity in the mind.

1 Stand in Mountain Pose (page 46). Lift the left heel up to rest at the top of the right thigh as you bend the supporting leg a little. Press the left knee toward the floor to open the right hip. Lengthen the tailbone toward the floor and elongate the spine.

2 On an inhalation, raise the arms above the head. On the exhalation, bring the palms of the hands together into the prayer position and lower the hands to rest in front of the heart center. Bend the right leg, lean forward more, and lift the

heart center as you sink down a little deeper into the squat. Keep the spine long, with the tailbone tucked under. The upper body will be leaning forward a little, but still vertical. Gaze at the fingertips of the hands, with your focus on softening and opening the heart. If you like, take your elbows to your shin.

3 Bring the spine more to vertical and bend the supporting knee more as you lift your left heel and lower yourself

INFORMATION

GAZE Tip of nose.

BUILD-UP POSES Tree Pose, Eagle Pose, Half Bound Lotus Stretch, Chair Pose.

COUNTER POSES Mountain Pose, Deep Forward Fold, Standing Splits, Standing Half Bow Balance.

LIGHTEN a) Stay at the first stage. **b)** Rest the lotus foot closer to the knee. **c)** Hold the raised foot in place with one hand.

EFFECT Focusing.

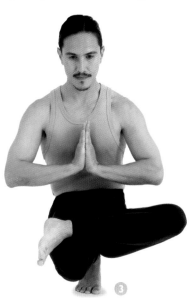

to a one-legged squat. Have the right hand between your sitting bones. Use your fingertips on the floor to help, if necessary, as you balance on the ball of your foot. Return the hands to the prayer position and take five steady breaths.

4 Take care as you come out of the pose. Inhale and raise yourself to standing. Release the lotus leg with control and return to Mountain Pose. Re-center yourself, then repeat on the other side.

Half Bound Lotus Stretch

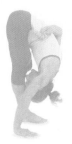

Ardha Baddha Padmottanasana

This pose massages the abdominal organs and improves the function of the large intestine. Tightness in the hips stresses the knees so care must be taken. To open the hips see Cow Posture (page 140) and Half Bound Lotus Forward Bend (page 146).

1 Stand in Mountain Pose (page 46). Inhale and lengthen the spine from the tailbone through to the base of the skull, then draw the crown of the head upward. Inhale and use your hands to lift the left foot up to the very top of the right thigh, so your left heel is just below the hip where the leg joins the trunk of the body. Press the inner left knee down and back, bringing the front of the thigh in line with the left hip.

INFORMATION

GAZE Tip of nose.

BUILD-UP POSES Cow Posture, Half Bound Lotus Forward Bend, Single Leg Forward Bend.

COUNTER POSES Chair Pose, Mountain Pose, Standing Half Bow

Balance, One Legged Sage Balance.

LIGHTEN a) Stay at the first stage.
b) Let the hands come to the floor if holding the foot from behind is difficult.

EFFECT Focusing.

2 Still holding the foot with your left hand, extend the left arm out to the side and behind to grasp the big toe of the left foot if possible. Inhale, extend the spine, and raise the right arm upward.

3 On the exhalation, fold forward from the hips, bringing the right hand to the floor beside the right foot. Allow the back of the neck to be long and the crown to come closer to the floor; move your forehead toward the knee. Inhale and lift the chest away from the thighs, looking forward and lengthening the spine from the sitting bones through to the base of the skull. Exhale and fold forward once again, releasing the spine and lengthening the whole front of the body along the upper thighs. Breathe smoothly and evenly, feeling the body stretch as you stay here.

4 Inhale and raise the right arm and spine up to standing. On the exhalation, release the left arm and return the left foot to stand in Mountain Pose. Repeat on the other side.

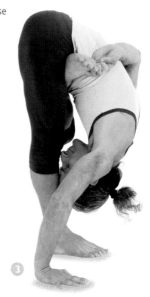

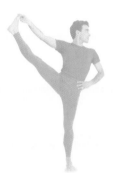

Upright
Big Toe Sequence

Hasta Padangusthasana This posture
limbers the hip joints, stretches the
hamstring muscles, tones the legs and
improves balance. It is part of the sequence
of standing postures in Ashtanga Vinyasa
Yoga (page 385).

1 Stand in Mountain
Pose (page 46).
Mentally take your
weight onto your left
leg. Press the left foot
down into the floor. Place
your left hand on your waist.
Your fingers pressing into
the abdomen will remind
you of Abdominal Lock
(page 338). Bend the right
knee and bring the right foot
up. Catch the big toe with the
index and the middle fingers

of the right
hand. Straighten
the right leg, stretching
the inner side of the foot
away. Keep the left leg straight
and active. Move the front of the left
thigh back and ground down with the sole
of the foot. Keep both hips an even height
from the floor. Hold for five breaths.

2 Still holding the toe, take the right
leg out to the side and turn the head
to look over the left shoulder. As in the
first position, keep the right hip down so

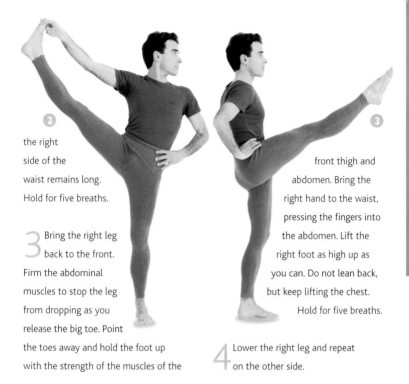

the right
side of the
waist remains long.
Hold for five breaths.

3 Bring the right leg
back to the front.
Firm the abdominal
muscles to stop the leg
from dropping as you
release the big toe. Point
the toes away and hold the foot up
with the strength of the muscles of the

front thigh and
abdomen. Bring the
right hand to the waist,
pressing the fingers into
the abdomen. Lift the
right foot as high up as
you can. Do not lean back,
but keep lifting the chest.
Hold for five breaths.

4 Lower the right leg and repeat
on the other side.

INFORMATION

GAZE Big toe and side.

BUILD-UP POSES Tree Pose, Deep
Forward Fold.

COUNTER POSES Standing Half
Bow Balance, Mountain Pose.

LIGHTEN a) Bend the knee and hold
it with one hand. **b)** Hold under the
thigh instead of the big toe. **c)** Bend
the knee while holding the big toe.
d) Grasp a belt looped around the ball
of the foot. **e)** Stand next to a wall to
help with your balance.

EFFECT Limbering.

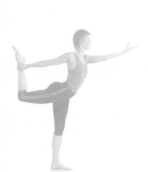

Standing
Half Bow Balance

Utthita Ardha Dhanurasana This
standing balance backbend enhances
the elasticity of the spine while toning
the abdominal organs and strengthening
the legs. The balance aspect is a
reminder that strength and grace
are possible at the same time.

1 Stand in Mountain Pose (page 46).
Inhale deeply onto the full length of
your body. Gradually transfer your weight
onto the left foot, and take your right
foot back to place the big toe on the floor
behind you. With hands on hips, lift out of
your lower back and arch your back into a
long backbend.

2 Bend the right knee and lift
the heel high in the air.
Stay in this backbend for a
few breaths to strengthen
the back muscles.

3 Bring the heel toward
the right buttock,
reach back with the right
hand, and grasp the outer
ankle with the right hand.
Press the right foot back
while you pull the ankle
forward with your right hand to
create as big an arch in your
"bow" as possible. Lift the right
leg backward to bring the thigh
more parallel to the floor and your
shin more vertical, sole of the foot
facing upward. Press your

right hip and right side ribs forward
to square your torso to the front.

4 Bend the supporting leg and lean
forward as you raise the left arm
parallel to the floor, palm facing up. Bring
the tips of the index
finger and thumb
together. With eyes soft,
gaze at the point of union
between the finger and thumb.
Breathe smoothly and evenly, balancing
with ease and grace on the left leg as the
right foot continues to push backward and

upward. Focus on
allowing the curve of
the spine to flow up
behind the heart as
you push the chest
open and keep the
shoulders even.

5 Release the right foot
as you exhale. Return to
stand evenly in Mountain Pose.
Repeat on the other side.

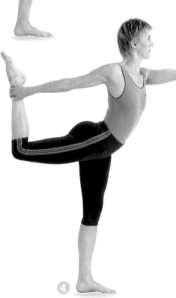

INFORMATION

GAZE Fingertips.

BUILD-UP POSES Warrior
Pose 3, Bow Pose, Single Leg
Swan Balance.

COUNTER POSES Restful Deep
Forward Fold, Single Leg
Forward Bend.

LIGHTEN a) Do not go to the
final stage. **b)** Practice near a wall
for balance.

EFFECT Focusing.

Dancer's Pose

Natarajasana This beautiful and very challenging posture requires balance and a high degree of flexibility in the back, legs, and shoulders. It is dedicated to Shiva the destroyer, the third god of the Hindu trinity, who is the Lord of the Dance.

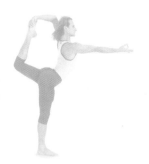

1 Stand in Mountain Pose (page 46). Lift the right foot off the floor, bring the knee back, and bend the right leg so that the sole of the foot is facing upward. Turn the toes out to the side, then reach back with the right hand and catch the inside of the right foot. Keep the standing leg straight and strong.

2 Rotate the elbow outward and upward (so you come to gripping the right big toe) while extending the right arm behind the head, at the same time bringing the right foot closer to the back of the head. Keep the right hip down as you are doing so and aim to have the right thigh parallel to the floor. Stretch the left arm out horizontally, palm facing down, and bring the tips of the left index finger and thumb together. This posture is Dancer's Pose 1 (the picture on the next page shows the pose on the left hand side of the body).

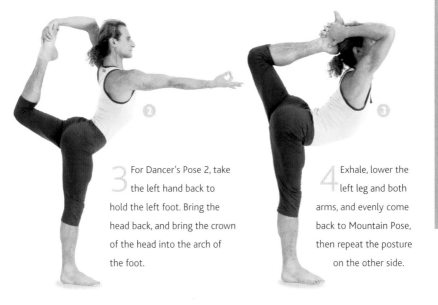

3 For Dancer's Pose 2, take the left hand back to hold the left foot. Bring the head back, and bring the crown of the head into the arch of the foot.

4 Exhale, lower the left leg and both arms, and evenly come back to Mountain Pose, then repeat the posture on the other side.

INFORMATION

GAZE At the tips of the front index finger and thumb in Dancer's Pose 1. Third eye in Dancer's Pose 2.

BUILD-UP POSES Lunges, Frog Pose, Standing Half Bow Balance, Pigeon Posture, Royal Pigeon Posture. Cow Posture opens the shoulders.

COUNTER POSES Standing Splits, Deep Forward Fold, Single Leg Forward Bend.

LIGHTEN a) Practice by lying on the floor, reaching the heel first to the buttock and then lifting the thigh off the floor, heel toward the head.
b) Stand in front of and about two feet from a wall and use it for balance.
c) Grasp a belt looped around the raised foot.

EFFECT Rejuvenating, energizing.

Seated & Floor Postures

The seated and floor postures help
loosen the body by releasing the
tension it holds so it can re-find its
balance. Forward bends tone the
abdominal organs and calm the nervous
system. They counter the ill effects of stress.
Folding yourself in a forward bend takes
the mind to a more receptive and
intuitive state. Then you can

listen to your heart.
With a quieter mind,
being fully supported by the
floor during seated postures
allows you to explore how you
yield to a posture. Rather than
force it, why not let
yourself release into
these postures?

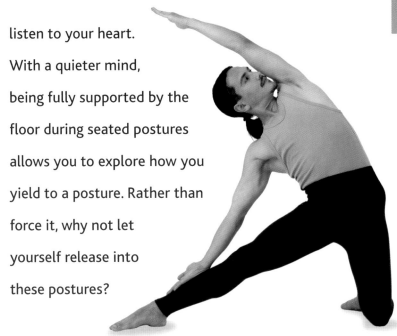

Child Pose

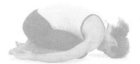

Balasana This restful posture restores balance and harmony to the body and puts the mind into an open and receptive state. Insert it into your practice in between other more demanding poses.

1 Kneel on the floor with the knees together. Let the buttocks rest down on the heels.

2 Lengthen upward through the spine. On an exhalation, tip forward from the pelvis to fold the upper body over so

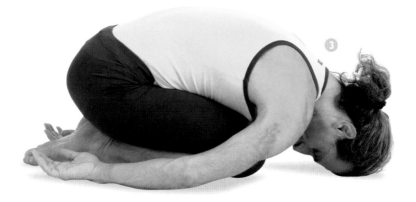

that the heart rests on top of the thighs and the forehead rests on the floor. Have the arms extended back beside the body, backs of the hands on the floor beside the feet, fingers curled softly. Let the upper back broaden as any tension drains away over the shoulders, down the arms, and out of the body. Relax your elbows completely. Melt away any tension in the neck. Relax and soften your lower back.

3 Child Pose offers us an opportunity to explore our breath. As the front of the torso releases to the thighs, chest and abdominal expansion is limited. Each time you inhale, tune into the movement of the breath in the back of the torso. Feel it widen and soften outward, all the way down to the sacrum. Each exhalation brings a sort of consolidation inward. Observe the flow of your natural breath through the whole body. Let the gentle pressure of the floor against your forehead allow the front of the brain to let go and relax deeply.

INFORMATION

GAZE Inward, eyes closed.

BUILD-UP POSE Yoga Seal Position.

COUNTER POSE East Stretch Posture, Locust Pose.

LIGHTEN a) Use a thinly folded blanket behind the knees. **b)** Pad under the tops of the feet if necessary. **c)** If your hips stay high in the air to give you an uncomfortable feeling of nose diving, rest your forehead on as many cushions as you need. Alternatively, rest your head on two stacked fists. **d)** If you are very flexible here and your neck feels as if it can't release properly, lay one or several layers of blanket across your thighs before laying your chest down to let your head hang down a little more.

EFFECT Centering.

Extended Child Pose

Utthita Balasana This extended version of Child Pose is a little more active than the original as it opens the shoulders and the chest and lets the breath move fully into the chest and belly.

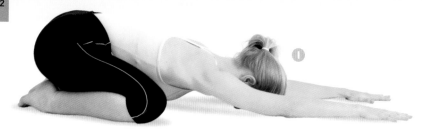

1 Kneel on the floor with the knees wide apart. The wider your knees, the deeper it will work into the hips. With big toes together, sit the buttocks back on the heels. Lengthen upward through the spine and, on an exhalation, slide the hands away to fold the upper body forward. Try to keep the buttocks in contact with the heels as you stretch forward through the hands—push back with the hands in the beginning to re-anchor your buttocks closer to the heels. Extend from the hips to the armpits, then lengthen from the armpits to the fingertips. Draw the shoulders down the back away from the ears and allow the back of the neck to be long, as your forehead rests down on the floor. As you hold the pose, tip your pelvis farther forward and let your side ribs release down between the inner thighs.

Embryo Pose

Pindasana We all have moments when life feels stressful, intense, and busy and demands more than we are able to give. At these times, it is useful to reconnect with the gentle aliveness that is always within us; it's just a matter of becoming quiet enough to be present with it.

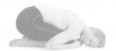

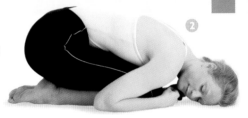

1 Be in Child Pose (page 100), kneeling on the floor with the upper body curled forward over the thighs. Allow the head to be turned to one side, with your cheek resting on the floor. Let the fingers curl very softly toward the palms. Nestle the fists between the chin and the knees.

2 Tune in to the soothing rhythm of the breath. Be nurtured by its gentle constancy. With your eyes closed, breathe gently into the heart center, allowing it to soften and rest more deeply down into your whole body with each breath. Stay here in this position for as long as you wish.

INFORMATION

GAZE Eyes closed, turning inward.

BUILD-UP POSES Child Pose, Yoga Seal Position.

COUNTER POSES East Stretch Posture, Locust Pose.

LIGHTEN See Child Pose.

EFFECT Soothing.

Seated Staff Posture

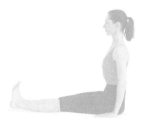

Dandasana This basic seated posture is the starting and finishing point of all sitting postures and twists. This posture awakens the entire body in preparation for more complicated asanas. It challenges us to pay attention to details.

1 Sit on the floor with your legs stretched out in front of you. Keep the big toes, inner heels, and inner knees together. Work your legs strongly by gripping the thigh muscles to the thigh bones and activating the muscles around the knee caps. Press the back of the knees into the floor. Make sure the legs do not rotate outward.

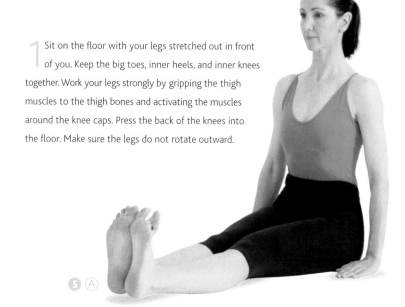

2 Move the heel bones and sitting bones away from each other by stretching the heels away from the body and tilting the pelvis slightly forward. You will have a feeling of lengthening the back of the legs as well as the lower back. It is important not to collapse the lower back, working strongly to lift from the base of the pelvis. Make sure your weight is equally distributed between the sitting bones.

3 Place the hands flat on the floor on either side of the hips with the fingers pointing forward. Allow your chest to lift, then broaden across the shoulders.

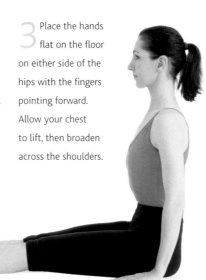

INFORMATION

GAZE Straight ahead with a level gaze.

BUILD-UP POSE Mountain Pose.

COUNTER POSE East Stretch Posture.

LIGHTEN a) Place a folded blanket under the sitting bones. **b)** Sit straight with your back against a wall, buttocks wedged as closely as possible against the wall.

EFFECT Calming.

4 Pull the navel in toward the spine, so you get a sense of lengthening the front of the torso. Having your tailbone act as a little anchor in this pose will let the rest of the vertebral column lift away from it, helping you sit long and tall.

5 Check the position of your head and neck. Have your chin parallel to the floor, which prevents the chin from jutting forward and helps maintain a nice length in the back of the neck. The pictures show a front-on view, Ⓐ and a side-on view. Ⓑ

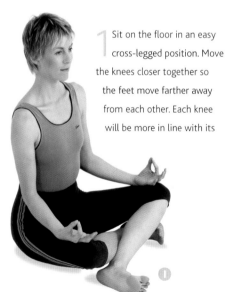

Easy Seated Pose

Sukhasana This simple seated posture opens the hips and abductor muscles of the thighs. If Lotus Posture (page 152) is not yet achievable for you, Easy Seated Pose is a comfortable position for meditation and pranayama.

1 Sit on the floor in an easy cross-legged position. Move the knees closer together so the feet move farther away from each other. Each knee will be more in line with its respective hip. Flex both feet, so the little toe sides of the feet contact the earth, rather than the tops of the feet. This position, with your shinbones parallel to each other, is more opening. If your knees are higher than your hip joints, you'll find it hard to sit with the spine erect. In this case, raise your seat with as many folded blankets as necessary.

2 To work deeper into the hips, come into Cross Legged Forward Stretch. Take your hands to the floor in front, inhale, and lengthen from your pubic bone

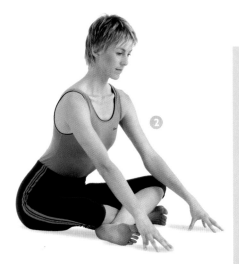

INFORMATION

GAZE Straight ahead when upright. Eyes closed when in forward bend.

BUILD-UP POSES Hip opening warm ups in Half Bound Lotus Forward Bend and Cow Posture, Cobbler's Pose, Reclining Bound Angle Pose.

COUNTER POSES Child Pose, Yoga Seal Position.

LIGHTEN Practice one leg at a time, seated on a chair.

EFFECT Centering.

to the base of the throat. Exhale and slide the hands away, maintaining the openness in the front of the trunk.

3 Keep the front edges of your sitting bones pressing into the floor and the heart lifted as you use the breath to

release and gradually walk the hands farther forward. Let the breath dissolve any holding around the hip socket as you stay for a minute or so. When you come up, change the crossing of the legs and repeat on the other side.

Toe Stretching Forward Bend

Utthita Anguli Sukhasana Most of us
live with our feet trapped inside shoes.
As a result, our feet are often less alive
than they could be. Enliven your toes by
stretching them out in this forward bend.
Let any other pose where you gaze at your
toes be a reminder to stretch them out.

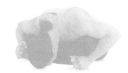

1 Sit in Easy Seated Pose (page 106) with
the left leg in front of the right. Lean
forward and use your right hand to help you
feed the fingers of your left hand in between
the toes of the right foot. Slide the fingers
as deeply in as possible.

2 Then, as best you can,
interlace the fingers of
your right hand with the
toes of the left
foot. Now gently
squeeze all
the toes.

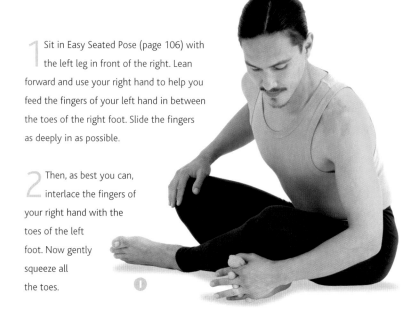

3 Flex the heels of the feet, fold forward and let the elbows move forward, like wings out to the sides of the body. On an exhalation, lengthen the upper body forward to bring the forehead to the floor. Stay for ten breaths, keeping both sitting bones on the floor, the front of the torso as long as the back of the torso. If it feels uncomfortable, use it as an opportunity to develop evenness of the mind in the face of adversity.

4 Inhale to come up, and release the hands. Cross the legs the other way, and repeat on the other side.

INFORMATION

GAZE Eyes closed or to tip of nose.

BUILD-UP POSE Easy Seated Pose.

COUNTER POSES Child Pose, East Stretch Posture.

LIGHTEN a) Simply wrap fingers around toes and squeeze them.
b) Raise the seat with cushions.
c) Remain upright.

EFFECT Extending, limbering.

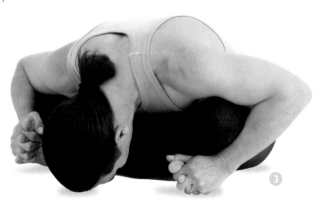

Lion Pose

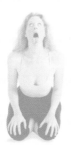

Simhasana This pose encourages us consciously to express the fierce side of ourselves! It activates the internal energy locks (bandhas) and clears the throat passage. It's a great exercise for the facial muscles, and its expressive nature leaves you feeling revived.

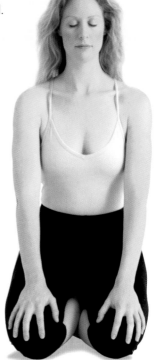

1 From a kneeling position, lean forward to lift the buttocks and cross your ankles. Have the left foot closest to the floor, with the toes of both feet pointing back. Drop the tailbone toward the floor and lengthen up through the spine.

2 Place the palms of the hands on the knees with the arms fully extended. Spread the fingers wide, fully energizing the arms from the shoulders through to the fingertips.

3 Close your eyes and take a long slow inhalation. On the exhalation, lean forward a little, open the jaw as wide as possible, and allow your tongue to roll out as far as it is able to reach. Aim to touch the chin. Roll your eyes back to gaze up at the third eye area which is in between the eyebrows. At the same time, as you exhale, make a roaring noise in the back of the throat. Hold this position and breathe through your mouth. Feel the skin on the face spread wide. Allowing our jaws to open this wide, combined with mouth breathing, can put us in touch with our animal nature.

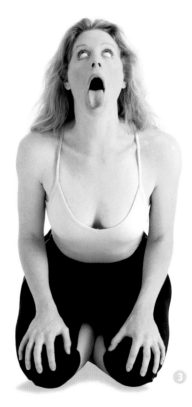

INFORMATION

GAZE Third eye.

COUNTER POSES Reclining Bound Angle Pose, Corpse Pose.

LIGHTEN a) Have a folded blanket under the ankles. **b)** Choose a simple kneeling position.

EFFECT Releasing.

4 Draw the tongue back inside the mouth, close the jaws and close the eyes. Sit quietly before beginning another round. Change the crossing of the legs to repeat twice more.

Perfect Pose

Siddhasana This pose increases the circulation in the lumbar spine and pelvic abdomen. It assists the mobility of the knee and ankle joints and is an excellent sitting posture for pranayama, chanting, or meditation.

1 Sit in Seated Staff Posture (page 104). Bend the right leg and bring the right heel to rest in toward the center line of the body. The sole of the right foot will be resting along the inner left thigh. Take the left heel to rest in front of the right ankle so it lies in front of the right heel.

2 Alternatively, you may fold the right leg in and press the heel against the perineum (the area between the anus and the genitals). Bring the sole and outer edge of the left foot to snuggle between the right calf muscle and the thigh. As your knees are wide and close to the floor, a solid foundation for sitting is established.

INFORMATION

GAZE Tip of nose/eyes closed gazing within.

BUILD-UP POSES Sitting still is easiest after warming the body with some general yoga postures.

COUNTER POSE Corpse Pose.

LIGHTEN a) Place the heel of the first leg at the center line of the body rather than the perineum. **b)** Sit on a folded blanket if the knees are far from the floor. **c)** Sit with your back against a wall.

EFFECT Meditative.

4 Draw the chin in toward the throat slightly so that the vertebrae of the neck flow on in a line from the spine. Have the eyes closed, or gaze softly at the tip of the nose. Stay here for some time, breathing deeply and gently through the whole body. Each time you practice Perfect Pose, alternate which leg you fold in first.

5 To practice Yoga Seal (see page 155), clasp one wrist with the other hand behind your back. Inhale, extend through the spine, then exhale and fold forward. If possible, bring the forehead to rest on the floor. This pose, which may also be practiced from a kneeling position, is a calming position and a suitable preparation for meditation.

3 Ground your weight down into both sitting bones and use this as the foundation to lengthen upward through the spine. With the arms extended and the elbows soft, allow the hands to rest lightly on top of the knees. Place your hands palms up or down or use a hand seal (*mudra*) of your choice.

Head Beyond the Knee Pose

Janu Sirsasana This pose tones the liver, spleen, and kidneys. Rather than aiming the head to the knee, creating a rounding of the back, aim to close the gap first between navel and thigh, then chest and thigh, and finally bringing the forehead to the shin.

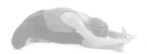

1 Sit on the floor in Seated Staff Posture (page 104). Bend the right knee out to the side. Keep a small gap between sole of the foot and the left thigh. Square both hips to the front.

2 Extend through the left heel. On an inhalation, raise the arms over the head. Rotate from the lower abdomen to turn your torso toward the left and line up your breastbone with the left thighbone. Keeping the spine long, exhale as you fold the upper body forward and grasp the left foot with both hands.

3 If you reach your foot, increase the challenge by taking the right knee back and as far out to the side as possible. In this position the top of your right

foot will come to the floor. Your right hip will be farther back than the left.

4 A more advanced variation is to sit on the heel of the bent leg. Place the heel under the perineum and, if possible, have the ankle hinge at a right angle. The toes point forward, rather than out to the side. When you combine it with the Great Lock (page 34) this creates a *mudra*, called Great Seal.

5 As you stay in the pose, keep moving the floating ribs forward.

Roll the shoulders away from the ears. Loop the hands around the sole of the foot, clasping the left wrist in the right hand. Bend the elbows. Press the back of the left knee to the floor. Stretch out the toes. Increase the intensity of the stretch in the right lower back by pressing the right thigh and knee to the floor. Stay for ten breaths or longer. Inhale to come up and repeat on the other side.

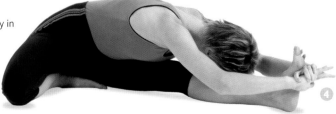

Revolved Head to Knee Pose

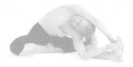

Parivrtta Janu Sirsasana Most of our day-to-day movements involve forward bending. This lateral stretch works into the tiny muscles between the side ribs while giving the torso a welcome twist.

1 Sit on the floor in Seated Staff Posture (page 104). Follow the steps for Head Beyond the Knee Pose (page 114) to bend and position the right leg. Raise the right arm out to the side and spiral from the shoulder to bring your palm to face backward. Turning from the lower abdomen, rotate your trunk to the right and wrap your arm behind your back to grasp your inner left thigh.

2 Reach your left arm in the air, extend from left hip to left armpit, and reach forward to grasp the inner left foot. Lengthen your side ribs along the left thigh. Move your right

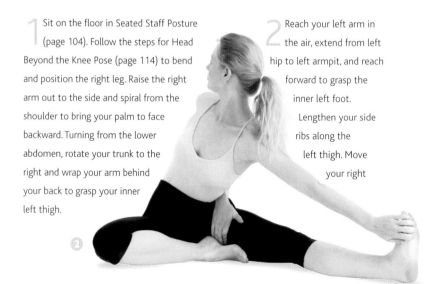

shoulder up and back to help fully open the chest toward the right.

3 Once you have sufficient flexibility, the left shoulder will press against the inner left knee. In the beginning, be satisfied to bring the elbow to the floor while holding the foot. Curve the left side ribs inward as you curve out the right side ribs and make the spine more of a "C" shape.

4 To continue to the second stage, turn the fingers and thumb of the left hand to face upward, still grasping the foot. Release the right hand from the thigh and take it overhead to hold the left toes. Move the right shoulder back so it is directly over the left shoulder. Bend the left elbow to bring your left shoulder closer to the floor. Press out through the right side of the trunk (so you curve it and the

INFORMATION

GAZE Upward.

BUILD-UP POSES Standing Side Stretch, Revolved Easy Pose Twist, Gate Pose, Seated Gate Pose.

COUNTER POSES East Stretch Posture, Double Leg Forward Stretch.

LIGHTEN a) Take the right hand to the sacrum or the floor behind. **b)** Take the left hand to grasp the thigh or shin. **c)** Use a belt to hold the extended foot.

EFFECT Centering.

spine away from the floor) to stretch the little muscles in between the right side ribs. Look up under the upper arm. Hold five to ten breaths, then repeat on the other side.

Double Leg Forward Stretch

Paschimottanasana The back of the body is given an intense stretch as the top half of the body folds over the bottom half. With the head tucked in, this pose offers an opportunity to reconnect deeply with our inner being.

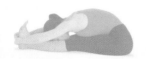

1 Sit in Seated Staff Posture (page 104) with palms or fingertips on the floor beside the hips. Tilt the pelvis anteriorly to tip your weight more onto the front edge of the sitting bones. The sitting bones anchor to the floor as you inhale and float the arms above the head. Let the heart lift and lengthen the spine up toward the crown of the head.

2 On an exhalation, gently draw the pubic abdomen in toward the spine as you fold the upper body forward,

extending the arms along the legs to hold the big toes or sides of the feet, or grasp one wrist around the balls of the feet.

3 Keeping the chest open, rather than rounding the upper back down, will help

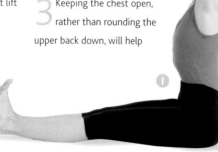

free up the breathing. On an inhalation, look forward, lift the heart center, and move the floating ribs away from the hips and toward the knees. This forward movement originates from the pelvic abdomen and lumbar spine rather than from the head and shoulders.

4 If you reach the feet easily, bend the elbows and exhale farther into the pose, bringing the forehead to the knees. If your chest is not close to the thighs, don't drop the head but keep the vertebrae of the neck in line with the rest of the vertebral column. Move your shoulders away from your ears.

5 When you reach your maximum extension in the pose, stay there breathing deeply for as long as you continue to enjoy the stretch. Keep the backs of the legs in full contact with the floor. Work to maintain the anterior tilt of the pelvis as the spine lengthens forward.

6 Release on an inhalation. Draw the lower abdominal area in toward the spine, raise the arms and chest upward. Lower the arms beside the hips on an exhalation, returning to Seated Staff Posture.

INFORMATION

GAZE Toes or third eye.

BUILD-UP POSES Seated Staff Posture, Cross Legged Forward Stretch, Deep Forward Fold, Head Beyond the Knee Pose.

COUNTER POSES Reclining Bound Angle Pose, East Stretch Posture, Locust Pose.

LIGHTEN a) Keep knees bent, see Restful Double Leg Forward Stretch. **b)** Bend knees and rest chest on thighs. **c)** Hold thighs or shins rather than feet.

EFFECT Calming.

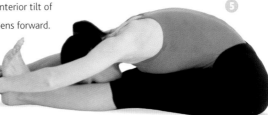

Hero Pose

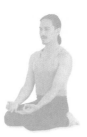

Virasana This kneeling seated pose stretches the front of the thighs and opens the ankle joints. As it reduces blood supply to the legs, it quiets the sensations of the body, so some find it useful for meditation. When you come out of Hero Pose, enjoy the rush of fresh blood to the knees.

1 Kneel on the floor with the feet wide apart and the knees as close together as possible. As you sit down between the feet, you may like to use your hands to roll the calf flesh externally and iron it down toward the heels so that the lower leg can snuggle more closely against the outer thigh. Have the tops of the feet on the floor. Your toes need to point backward in this pose, never out to the sides, which would place the inner knee at risk. Have the thigh bones parallel.

2 Hold the big toe of each foot with the thumb and index finger, and separate the big toe from the second toe. Continue down, spreading all of the toes apart and widening the soles of the feet.

2 Let your sitting bones come easily to the floor. From this well-grounded foundation, sit tall and draw the lower abdomen in toward the spine to get the sensation of the spine lengthening

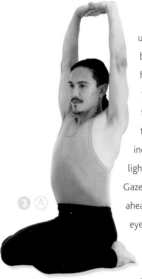

upward. Rest the backs of the hands on top of the knees, with the tip of the thumb and index fingers lightly touching. Gaze softly straight ahead or, with the eyes closed, focus on the space between the eyebrows. Stay here for as long as you enjoy deepening into your own being.

INFORMATION

GAZE Tip of nose.

BUILD-UP POSES One Leg Folded Forward Bend, Child Pose.

COUNTER POSES Reclining Bound Angle Pose, Head Beyond the Knee Pose, Seated Staff Posture, East Stretch Posture.

LIGHTEN a) Bring the big toes together to sit on the heels. **b)** Sit on a bolster. **c)** Widen the knees slightly. **d)** Have a folded blanket to pad under the inner ankles. **e)** Place a thin layer of fabric in the back of the knees.

EFFECT Centering.

3 Once you wish to release from the pose, inhale and raise the hands above the head. With the arms stretching fully away, interlace the fingers and extend the palms toward the ceiling. This is Mountain Pose 2 . When you release the arms, allow the palms to rest lightly on the heels of the feet and fold the upper body forward, perhaps bringing the forehead to rest on the floor. Then kneel up onto all fours.

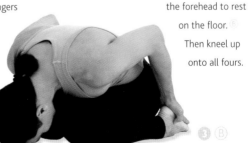

One Leg Folded Forward Bend

Trianga Mukhaikapada Paschimottanasana This pose stretches the hamstring muscle and limbers the knees and ankle. It is recommended for easing sciatica. Like most forward bends, it tones the digestive organs.

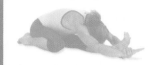

1 Sit in Seated Staff Posture (page 104), pressing the backs of the knees strongly to the floor.

2 Bend the right knee and bring the right foot beside the right hip. Lean to the left and take your right thumb to the top of your calf muscles. Use the thumb to roll the calf flesh out to the right, and iron it down toward the heel. Have the toes pointing straight back or slightly inward, with the tops of both the big and little toes touching the floor. Take care here, because having the toes pointing outward puts the knee at risk. Keep the thighbones parallel so the right knee is fairly close to the left knee.

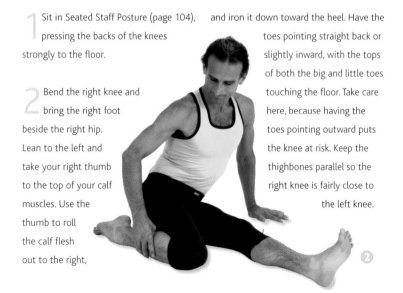

3 Press down well through the right buttock so that your weight feels equally distributed between the sitting bones. If the right ankle hurts at this stage, practice Hero Pose (page 120).

4 Inhale and lengthen the front of the body. Let the chest lift as you draw in the area of the abdomen below the navel. Exhale and fold forward, keeping this length in the front of the torso. Hold the right wrist with the left hand beyond the foot. Rest the forehead or chin on the left shin beyond the knee.

5 Unhunch and broaden the shoulders so they feel relaxed even as they are working for you. Re-anchor well through the right sitting bone. Deepen the pose by bringing your chest forward and down. Hold for ten breaths.

INFORMATION

GAZE Big toe.

BUILD-UP POSES Hero Pose, Double Leg Forward Stretch.

COUNTER POSES Cat Pose, East Stretch Posture.

LIGHTEN a) Place a folded blanket or a block under the left buttock bone. **b)** Place some padding under the top of the foot of the bent leg. **c)** Bend the knee of the leg extended out in front. **d)** Use a strap around the ball of the front foot.

EFFECT Calming, grounding.

6 Come up on an inhalation, then exhale and straighten the right leg to come back to Seated Staff Posture. Repeat on the other side.

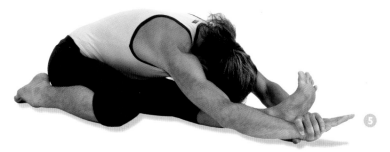

Heron Posture

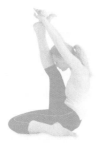

Krounchasana The extended leg resembles the neck and head of a bird in this posture. It stretches the hamstring muscles and limbers the hips, knees, and ankles. It is similar to the Three Limbed Forward Stretch, just in a different relationship to gravity.

1 Sit in Seated Staff Posture (page 104). Bend the left knee and bring the left foot beside the

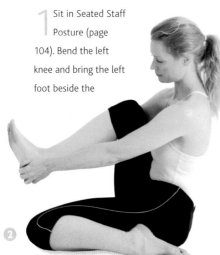

left hip with the toes pointing straight back or slightly inward, but *not* outward. Lean to the right and take your left thumb to the top of your calf muscles. Use the thumb to roll the calf flesh out to the right and iron it down toward the heel. Sit erect once again and press down through the right sitting bone to keep the weight equally distributed between both buttocks. The top of the big and little toes should both be touching the floor, the knees just a couple of inches (a few centimeters apart). If the right ankle hurts at this stage, practice Hero Pose (page 120) and One Leg Folded Forward Bend (page 122) before learning this pose.

2 Bend the right knee and bring it close to the trunk. Hold the right heel with both hands. Straighten the right leg vertically. While doing so use your hands to press down on the heel as if you want to shorten the distance between the right heel and right sitting bone. While it might seem contradictory, this actually helps the leg to straighten.

3 Adhere the right thigh muscles to the thighbone and open the back of the right knee, keeping the right leg (the neck of the heron) straight and long. Lifting from the tailbone, curve in the lower back and slowly bring the chin to the right shin, looking up toward your right foot. If possible, grasp the left wrist with the right hand. Don't round the back or collapse the chest. Keep the right leg centered. Stay for ten breaths.

4 Exhale, bring the right leg down, and straighten the left leg, then repeat on the other side.

INFORMATION

GAZE Toes.

BUILD-UP POSES Hero Pose and One Leg Folded Forward Bend, Double Leg Forward Stretch.

COUNTER POSES Cobbler's Pose, East Stretch Posture.

LIGHTEN a) Do not go to the final stage. **b)** Use a belt around the foot and/or bend the raised leg. **c)** Place some padding under the top of the foot of the bent leg.

EFFECT Challenging, calming.

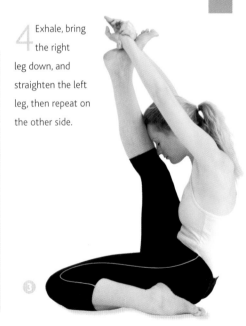

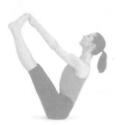

Double Toe Hold

Ubhaya Padangusthasana This pose
has effects similar to those of Double
Leg Forward Stretch (page 118), with
the additional challenge of balancing.

1 Sit in Seated Staff
Posture (page 104) with the
legs extended. Bend the knees and
bring the heels close to the buttocks.
Hold each big toe between the thumb
and forefinger. On an exhalation,
straighten the legs upward, so you are
balancing on the buttocks. Press the sitting
bones into the floor and draw the pubic
abdomen in toward the spine. Avoid
collapsing the ribs into the belly—move
the lower back in and lift the chest toward
the knees as you lengthen the spine. Keep
the back of the legs long, extending

through the
heels. Move your
face toward the sky,
maintaining the length
in the back of the neck.

2 If you are comfortable there, this
pose can be extended just as in
Double Leg Forward Stretch by interlacing
the fingers around the soles of the feet.
Stay here for several breaths before
coming out of the posture.

INFORMATION

GAZE Third eye.

BUILD-UP POSES Boat Pose, Double Leg Forward Stretch, Heron Posture, Half Lotus Heron Pose.

COUNTER POSES Corpse Pose, East Stretch Posture.

LIGHTEN a) Keep the knees bent, with the forearms folded behind them. **b)** Use a strap around the balls of the feet. **c)** Grasp heels instead of toes and pull back firmly on them as you straighten the legs and torso. **d)** Practice with your back or toes against a wall.

EFFECT Focusing.

3 A further extension of this pose is Upward Facing Forward Balance. From a seated position, raise the legs up. Bend the knees so the shins are parallel to the floor. Place your forearms along the calves, fingers cupping heels. Keep your abdomen and thighs snugly close. Ⓐ On an exhalation, straighten the legs while pulling back on the heels with the fingers. Close the gap between your chest and thighs. Draw your face toward your shins. Open the backs of your knees to straighten them fully. This pose can also become a *mudra*, the Seal of Thunderbolt. Ⓑ To evolve this position to a *mudra* practice The Great Lock (page 341). On an exhalation, release the hands and legs back to the floor to lie resting in Corpse Pose (page 310).

Ⓑ Ⓐ Ⓑ Ⓑ

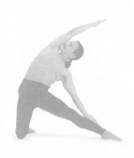

Gate Pose

Parighasana The unusual shape of this pose invites us to open our view of who we are and what shape we make in the world. As we practice both sides, we improve the circulation of prana, our vital energy.

1 Kneel and step the left foot out to the side with the left heel in line with the right knee. Keep your front thigh muscles active as you press the left toes down to the floor. Raise the right arm overhead as you inhale. Turn the palm of the hand up. Tuck the tailbone under and lengthen up through the spine.

2 Move the left hip forward to bring it directly above the knee. On the exhalation, curve inward deeply at the left waist and extend the left arm along the front of the left leg, palm still facing up. Resist the temptation to lean forward—keep the back of the body on one plane.

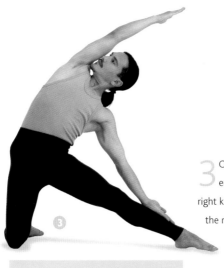

③ On an inhalation, lift through the entire length of the right side from right knee to fingertips. Exhale and arch the right arm over the head toward the left foot. Maintain an openness in the right armpit by easing the right arm back so your shoulders are one above the other. Bring the palms of the hands toward each other and turn the head to gaze upward from under the right arm. Stay here for a few breaths, feeling the upper ribs expand.

④ Release the right arm on an inhalation, raising the trunk back to the center. Return the left leg to kneeling. Close your eyes and take some breaths while you experience the subjective difference in length between your right and left sides. Then repeat on the other side.

INFORMATION

GAZE Upward past underarm.

BUILD-UP POSES Standing Side Stretch, Revolved Head to Knee Pose, Seated Gate Pose.

COUNTER POSES East Stretch Posture, Double Leg Forward Stretch, Downward Facing Dog Pose.

LIGHTEN a) Press right palm to thigh for support. **b)** Keep left hand on hip or extend it vertically upward. **c)** Practice cross-legged.

EFFECT Releasing.

Seated Angle Posture

Upavista Konasana This posture stretches the inner thighs, tones the legs, opens the hips, and stimulates the blood flow in the pelvic region. It is one of the most useful for gynecological problems because it regulates the menstrual flow and ovarian function. It is a good pose to practice during menstruation and pregnancy.

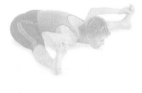

1 Sit in Seated Staff Posture (page 104). Spread the legs wide apart. Press the back of the knees into the floor to energize the legs and ensure the knees and toes face straight up, rather than rolling in or out. Place the hands on the floor beside the hips. Stretch the heels away from the hips to straighten and lengthen the back of the legs. Lift up the chest and roll the pelvis forward to increase the inward curve of the lower back. Hold for a few breaths.

2 Exhale, lean forward, and catch the big toes with the index and middle fingers, arms straight. While it is easy to feel how the back of the torso lengthens in

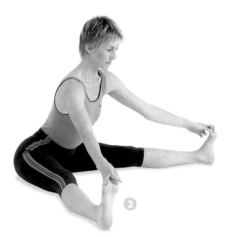

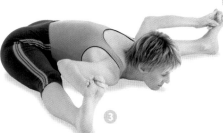 Exhale and extend the chest farther
forward as you lower it down. Rest
the forehead, or if possible, the chin and
the chest on the floor. Stretch the hands
away to broaden the chest. Keep the toes
and knees pointing upward. Breathe
softly and steadily and be patient as
you surrender deeper into the posture.
To come out of the pose, use your hands
to support under your knees as you bring
the legs back together.

this position, the challenge of this posture
is to keep lengthening the front of the
torso. Pull the navel in toward the
spine on each inhalation (see
Abdominal Lock, page 338) and
avoid rounding the back. Pull up
strongly with the muscles of the front
thighs. Hold for a few more breaths.

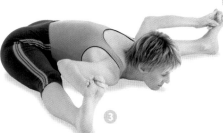

INFORMATION

GAZE Forward and up.

BUILD-UP POSES Head Beyond the
Knee Pose, Double Leg Forward
Stretch, Wide Leg Forward Bend.

COUNTER POSES Cobbler's Pose,
Cow Posture, East Stretch Posture.

LIGHTEN a) Do not go to the final
stage. **b)** Use belts around the feet, or
grasp higher up on the legs. **c)** Sit on a
folded blanket and/or have your back
against a wall.

EFFECT Calming.

Seated Side Stretch Sequence

Parsva Upavista Konasana The sideways stretch counters stiffness in the back and welcomes a loose fluidity into the body. The twisted version releases the lower back in a similar way to Head Beyond the Knee Pose (page 114).

1 Sit with your legs wide apart. Have your kneecaps and toes facing straight upward. Extend through your heels and turn your toes back toward your torso. Take your fingertips to the floor behind you. Take several breaths to float your torso up out of your hips. Rather than growing taller from a hard, teeth-gritted attitude, let it be effortless and joyful.

2 Once you have a sense of freeing up and elongation, reach your left arm up in the air. Take your right hand to the right thigh. On an exhalation, make a long deep curve from your left hip to the heel of the left hand as you fold to the right. Curve in deeper along the right side of the torso, and round out the left side more, as if you wanted the left side ribs to touch the side wall. This pushing out with the left side ribs gives a sense of lightness to the posture.

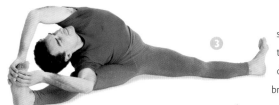

3 If you are more flexible, both hands might hold the foot. Take care not to insist you reach your foot at the expense of flattening out and losing the curves in your sides. Keep your left shoulder over your right, not forward of it. Anchor your left sitting bone to the floor. Extend the line of energy from left hips to left hand. Hold for five to ten breaths.

so it is above your thigh. Let the left lower back lengthen diagonally as you line up your breastbone with your right leg. Lower your left shoulder and arm to bring them level with the right. Grasp the ball of your foot. Spread some mental energy to your left leg. Press the back of the leg evenly to the floor and extend through the heel. Draw in the navel with each inhalation. Let your floating ribs move closer to your knee with each exhalation. On every exhalation feel your waist narrowing as you twist more. Take five or ten long breaths. Then repeat on the other side.

4 Now bring a twist into your posture, rotating from your lower abdomen and turning your navel

INFORMATION

GAZE Tip of nose.

BUILD-UP POSES Revolved Easy Pose, Seated Gate Pose, Head Beyond the Knee Pose, Seated Angle Posture.

COUNTER POSES Cobbler's Pose,

Cow Posture.

LIGHTEN a) Bend the right knee.
b) Side Stretch—stay at Stage 2.
c) Twist—grasp the thigh or calf.

EFFECT Limbering.

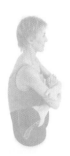

Cobbler's Pose

Baddha Konasana This seated pose strongly stretches the adductor muscles of the inner thighs. Anyone with tight hips will benefit from daily practice of this posture. Because of the focus on the perineal floor, the organs of the entire pelvic region are toned and invigorated by the practice of this pose.

1 From Seated Staff Posture (page 104) bend the knees out to the side and bring the soles of the feet together. Draw the legs toward the body and snuggle the heels into the perineum.

2 Let your fingertips cup the floor behind the back. Press down strongly into the sitting bones as you lengthen upward through the spine and lift the heart center. Bring your attention to the inner edge of both thighs. Lengthen outward toward the inner knees, as if trying to touch the side walls with the knees. This will assist the movement of the knees closer to the floor. Allow some long exhalations to soften any tension in the inner thighs—you cannot force this stretch to happen. It is simply a matter of surrendering and allowing!

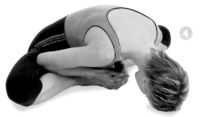

4 Now bring the elbows to the inner thighs and press down as you fold the upper body forward. Keep the front of the body long as you bring your forehead to the floor.

3 If your sense of "sitting tall" feels well established, hold the feet with both hands. Use the thumbs to move the big toes apart and spread the soles of the feet wide, so they open out like a book. This helps the knees ease toward the floor. Alternatively, work on assisting the torso to float up out of the hips by interlacing your fingers around the feet and lengthening the sides of the waist upward.

5 A balancing version of Cobbler's Pose is Navel Pressure Pose. Cup your feet and lift them in the air. Lift them up as high as possible, then work the big toes toward your chest. While the feet move toward your body, the knees press back. If possible, wrap the forearms farther around to grasp the elbows.

INFORMATION

GAZE Tip of nose or straight ahead.

BUILD-UP POSES Reclining Bound Angle Pose, Head Beyond the Knee Pose, Extended Child Pose, Garland Pose, preparations for Lotus Posture.

COUNTER POSES Seated Angle Posture, Hero Pose, East Stretch Posture.

LIGHTEN a) Sit with the back against a wall. **b)** Sit on a bolster or folded blanket to raise the seat. **c)** Use a weight like a sandbag on top of each thigh.

EFFECT Opening.

Reclining Bound Angle Pose

Supta Baddha Konasana This pose gently opens the hips and the adductor muscles of the inner thighs. It eases many digestive and reproductive disorders because the pelvis benefits from a steady supply of blood. This version opens the chest and encourages steady breathing.

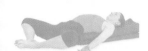

1 Sit on the floor in Seated Staff Posture (page 104). Have the narrow end of a bolster or the short edge of one to three folded blankets against the sacrum. Bring the soles of the feet together, widen the knees apart, and draw the heels up to rest against the perineum. You may wish to use a soft belt (or bathrobe tie) to hold the feet in position and place a pleasurable traction through the sacrum. If so, loop the belt around the outside of the feet, run it up the insides of the knees and around the lower back. When you are sitting up, the strap will sit just off the inner thighs. Keep it loose, and tighten it up fully only after lying back.

2 Lie back, vertebra by vertebra, until you are lying flat. The buttocks are in full contact with the floor, with the upper body fully supported by the bolster. You may find you can draw the heels closer to the body and tighten the belt further. Check that the back of the neck is in line with the spine, chin tucked in toward the chest. You may be most comfortable with a small support under the head to bring it higher than your heart. If you like, use an eye pillow.

3 Allow the arms to rest beside the body and close the eyes, bringing your attention deeply within your own being. Allow the belly to be soft. Relax any holding in the hip sockets as you surrender and open your inner thighs to the gentle force of gravity. Stay here for five to ten minutes, breathing smoothly and evenly.

4 The following option is more easily accessible during your practice. Lie on the floor in Corpse Pose (page 310). Bring the soles of the feet together by the groin and drop the knees out to the side. Experiment to find the best heel/groin distance for your body. Rest with the arms relaxed beside the body. Allow the back of the neck to be long, with the chin tucked in toward the chest.

INFORMATION

GAZE Internal.

BUILD-UP POSE Extended Child Pose.

COUNTER POSES Child Pose, Hero Pose.

LIGHTEN a) Support under each knee with folded blankets. **b)** Lie back over a higher support.

EFFECT Nourishing.

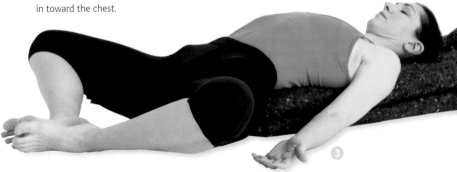

Garland Pose

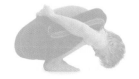

Malasana This deep squat with the feet together is extremely beneficial for the muscles, organs, and soft tissue of the pelvic abdomen. The legs are enlivened, the hips opened, and the lumbar spine is given a supported stretch. This simple pose is often an unexpected challenge for Westerners who are generally not used to squatting.

1 Stand with the feet hip width apart and fold forward to a wide stance Restful Deep Forward Fold (page 313). Turn the toes out, bend the knees, lift the heels and lower the buttocks toward the floor to a deep squat. Take the knees wide apart, so they track over the toes.

2 Reach the hands forward to touch the floor. Use the fingers on the floor to help take weight through the pelvis to let the hips drop back. Then lower the heels closer to the floor.

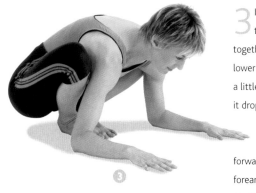

3 If your heels come close to, or touch the floor, bring the feet closer together so the big toes touch and again lower the heels to floor. Imagine you have a little weight tied to the tailbone to help it drop closer to the floor. Fold forward and, if possible, bring your forearms to the floor, fingers pointing forward. If that is easy, then drape your forearms along the floor under the legs so the fingers point back. Then grasp the heels and fold your trunk farther forward.

INFORMATION

GAZE Tip of nose.

BUILD-UP POSES Cobbler'sPose, Seated Angle Posture, Head Beyond the Knee Pose.

COUNTER POSES Hero Pose, Seated Staff Posture, East Stretch Posture.

LIGHTEN a) Stay at an earlier stage. Use a folded blanket under the heels. **b)** Use a strap for your hands behind the back.

EFFECT Centering.

4 For the full pose, internally rotate the shoulders to take one arm at a time under the shins and bring the back of the hand to the sacrum. Grasp the fingers. Soften your heels to the floor. Soften your self-criticism. Be content with whichever version you arrive at as you hold for five to ten breaths.

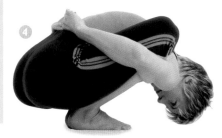

Cow Posture

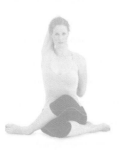

Gomukhasana Looking at it from above, this posture resembles the face of a cow, with the feet making the horns and the knees making the mouth. Many find they need practice to bring the feet in a symmetrical position to look like a cow and not a unicorn! This posture limbers the hips and legs, as well as the shoulders.

1 Many people benefit by first warming up the hips with Ankle to Knee Pose. Sit cross-legged with the left leg in front. Pick up the left leg and place the left ankle on top of the right knee. Position the lower leg so the right ankle is on the floor underneath the left knee and the shinbones will form a triangle with the thighs. Flex the heels of both feet, activating the inner thigh and calf muscles. Let gravity help the left knee release down. To increase the hip opening, lean forward and slide the hands along the floor. Stay for one minute, then change sides.

2 Sit on the floor with the feet apart and the knees slightly bent. Bring the right foot under the left knee and place the heel close to the left hip. Have the toes pointing left. Then bring the left foot close to the right hip, toes pointing to the right. The left knee

should now be over the right knee. If it doesn't approach this, work on hip openers, such as preparation for Cow Posture (page 140) and Half Bound Lotus Forward Bend (page 146). Keep the weight equally distributed between the sitting bones. Press the left knee down with both hands to bring the knees together.

3 Extend your left arm out to the side, and rotate the shoulder inward so the palm faces back and thumb points down. Bend the elbow and bring the left hand behind the back, palm facing outward. Stretch the right arm up, spiral the arm from the shoulder so that the thumb points backward, then bend the elbow to clasp the hands behind the back. Move the right elbow back and more to the center line behind the head and lift the chest. Front view, Ⓐ back view. Ⓑ Release the hands, then the legs, and repeat on the other side.

INFORMATION

GAZE Upward.

BUILD-UP POSES Easy Seated Pose Forward Bend, Half Lotus Pose, Cow Face Forward Fold.

COUNTER POSES Hero Pose, Extended Child Pose, Seated Staff Posture.

LIGHTEN a) Sit on a block or folded blanket. **b)** Hold a belt between the hands and inch the hands together.

EFFECT Centering.

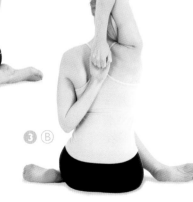

Cow Face Forward Fold

Gomukha Paschimottanasana It feels impossible to "cheat" in this pose. Pressing down on the thigh with the top leg stops any unconscious bending of the knee and increases the intensity of the pose. The position of the arms minimizes any rounding of the back and keeps the muscles of the upper spine working.

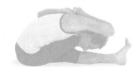

1 From Seated Staff Posture (page 104), bend your right leg and take it across the left thigh so the right toes point out to the side. Your right knee will be stacked on top of the left.

2 Raise the right arm up high. Loosen the shoulder joint, and rotate the shoulder internally so that the little fingers turn to the front. Bend the elbow to bring the right hand down between the shoulder blades.

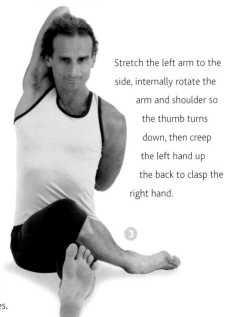

Stretch the left arm to the side, internally rotate the arm and shoulder so the thumb turns down, then creep the left hand up the back to clasp the right hand.

3

3 Lift the head and draw the chin in
toward the throat, keeping the back
of the neck long. Lift the heart as you
open the upper elbow toward the ceiling
and behind the head so it comes more to
the center line of the body.

4 Sit tall. Lift the torso out of the pelvis.
If you are comfortable here, on an
exhalation, draw the pubic abdomen in
toward the spine as you lengthen the front
of the body along the legs and fold the
upper body forward. Aim to land your
floating ribs beyond your upper knee. Use
your abdominal muscles to draw you
farther forward and down. Stay here for
five breaths, opening the shoulders as you
extend forward. The position of the arms
has trained your back to stay relatively

INFORMATION

GAZE Front toes.

BUILD-UP POSES Double Leg
Forward Stretch, Cow Posture,
Cross Legged Forward Stretch,
Seated Half Spinal Twist, hip
opening exercise from Half Bound
Lotus Forward Bend.

COUNTER POSES East Stretch
Posture, Locust Pose.

LIGHTEN a) Let the top knee be in
the air, sole of the foot on the
ground. **b)** Don't fold forward.
c) Walk your hands together
grasping a soft belt.

EFFECT Opening.

straight. Now, without rounding the back,
release the arms, grasp the front foot or
leg and lever yourself into a deep forward
bend. On an inhalation, raise the
upper body and release the arms
overhead. Lower the arms
on an exhalation and
return to Seated Staff
Posture. Repeat on the
other side.

Sage Forward Bend A

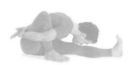

Marichyasana A This posture stretches the hamstrings, opens the hips, and stimulates the blood flow in the pelvic and abdominal region.

1 Sit in Seated Staff Posture (page 104). Bend the right knee up and bring the right heel in front of the right sitting bone, so the toes point straight forward. Have 2–3 inches (5–8 centimeters) between the right foot and the inner left thigh. Take a few attempts to pull the shin closer in, each time wedging the heel a little closer to the buttock.

2 Press down on the floor with the left hand behind you to help the pelvis tip forward. You may even be able to lift your buttocks off the floor to assist this tilting action. Reach the right arm past the inner right leg to bring the right armpit against the right shin. Rotate the right shoulder inward so the thumb turns in and down to the floor.

3 Then bring the hand back, wrapping the arm around the bent knee. With your right arm locked in place, lower both buttocks to the floor.

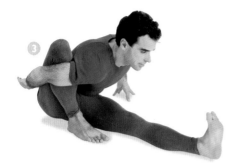

4 Reach the left arm forward, internally rotate the shoulder and take the arm around and behind to grasp the left wrist in your right hand. Exhale, lengthen the front of the body, bend forward and lengthen the floating ribs away from the hipbones and down. Extend the crown of the head toward the toes and let the chin come to the left shin. Keep the left leg energized, with the left knee and

toes facing upward rather than pointing out to the side. Press the back of the left leg against the floor. Press the sole of the right foot to the floor, and work the leg as if it was wanting to help you stand up. Keep the shoulders parallel to the floor and extend both wrists away from your back, as if to straighten the arms. Stay for ten breaths or more. Exhale, release the hands and come to Seated Staff Posture before repeating on the other side.

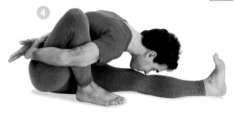

INFORMATION

GAZE Toes.

BUILD-UP POSES Head Beyond the Knee Pose, Double Leg Forward Stretch, Bound Sage Pose.

COUNTER POSE East Stretch Posture.

LIGHTEN a) Use a belt to link the hands behind the back. **b)** Do not go to the forward bending stage. **c)** It is also possible to make this a twisting posture by twisting the trunk to the left (away from the bent knee), instead of bending forward.

EFFECT Calming, anchoring.

Half Bound Lotus Forward Bend

Ardha Baddha Padma Paschimottanasana This forward bend opens the hips and knees and stretches the spine. The abdominal organs are toned as circulation to the pelvis is increased. The position of the heel also benefits the digestive system.

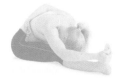

1 Many people find it useful to warm up the hips first by cradling one leg to the chest. Hold the knee and foot and press them together, or if you have the ability, take the foot and knee in the crook of your elbows and interlace your fingers. Then work into the hip joint by moving your bent leg slowly from side to side. Unhurriedly, take your hip through its full range of motion. Repeat on the other side.

2 Sit on the floor with both legs extended in Seated Staff Posture (page 104). Bend the left knee as in the warm up position. To bring the leg into Half Lotus Pose (page 152), hold the left foot in close to the navel and let the left knee move forward as it moves down toward the earth (so there is a sense of rolling the ball of the thighbone in the hip socket while you square the hips to the front.)

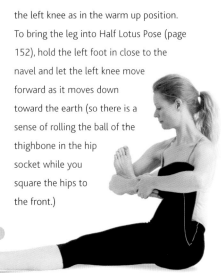

INFORMATION

GAZE Front toes or tip of nose.

BUILD-UP POSES Reclining Cobbler's Pose, Head Beyond the Knee Pose, Garland Pose, Cow Posture.

COUNTER POSES One Leg Folded Forward Bend, East Stretch Posture,

LIGHTEN a) Practice only the first stage. **b)** Don't wrap the arm around the body. **c)** Grasp a belt looped around the outstretched foot and/or the ankle of the bent knee. **d)** Bring the extended arm just to the knee. **e)** Place sole of foot of the bent leg on the floor instead of on the top of the thigh.

EFFECT Calming.

3 Bring the outer ankle to the very top of the right thigh. If the outer edge of the left foot is all that reaches the thigh you risk overstretching the ligaments, so it is best to work on hip opening poses to build toward this pose at a later stage.

4 On an exhalation, twist the torso to the left, rotate the left shoulder inward, and reach the left forearm behind the waist to grasp the toes of the left foot with the fingers of the left hand.

5 Create length in the spine before folding the upper body forward from the hips, bringing the chest toward the right thigh and clasping the right foot with the right hand. Grasp the big toe of the left foot with the thumb and forefinger of the left hand.

6 Stay here for five to ten breaths. Continue to move the chest forward, opening the heart as you draw the shoulder blades down the back. Lengthen the front of the body. Inhale to come up and repeat on the other side.

Sage Pose B

Marichyasana B This posture stretches
the hamstrings, opens the hips, and
stimulates the blood flow in the pelvic
region. Due to the pressure of the heel
on the abdomen, it stimulates the
digestive organs.

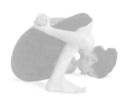

1 Sit in Seated
Staff Posture
(page 104). Bend
the left knee and
bring the foot as far up
as possible on the right
thigh, into Half Lotus
Pose (page 152). For preparations for
this position (Half Lotus Pose), see Half
Bound Lotus Forward Bend (page 146).

2 Then bend the right knee and bring
the right foot in front of the right
sitting bone, with the sole of the foot

pressing against the floor and the
toes pointing straight forward.
Leave 2–3 inches (5–8
centimeters) between the
right foot and the
inner left thigh.
Exhale and reach
the right arm
forward past
the inner right thigh. Rotate the shoulder
internally so the elbow points upward.
Move the right side ribs beyond the inner
thigh by pressing the left hand to the floor
behind you to maximize this forward lean.

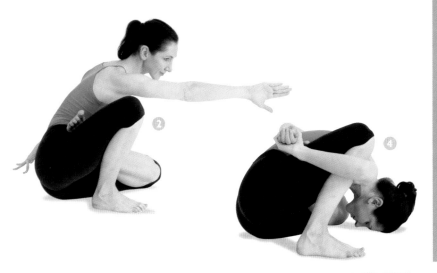

3 Take the right hand to the right, wrapping the arm around the bent knee. Reach behind your back with your left hand and clasp the left wrist.

4 Exhale and bend forward, bringing the forehead toward the floor. Keep the shoulders parallel to the floor. Keep the front of the torso long and the back straight. Reach the wrists away from the back and lift them up. Stay for ten breaths or more.

5 Exhale, release the hands, sit up, straighten the legs, then repeat on the other side.

INFORMATION

GAZE Tip of nose.

BUILD-UP POSES Sage Forward Bend A, Half Lotus Pose, Half Bound Lotus Forward Bend.

COUNTER POSE East Stretch Posture.

LIGHTEN a) Do not go to the final stage. **b)** Use a belt to link the hands behind the back. **c)** Instead of binding hands behind the back, hold the right knee with both hands and simply sit up straight.

EFFECT Calming.

Toe Stretching Head Beyond the Knee Pose

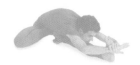

Janu Sirsasana C This posture works the toe joints, hips, and knees strongly. It also stretches the hamstrings and Achilles tendons and tones the abdominal organs.

1 Sit in Seated Staff Posture (page 104). Bend the right knee and take hold of the right heel with the left hand and the right toes with the right hand. (Have your right forearm between your right thigh and the calf.) Place the toes in front of the perineum, pulling the toes toward the

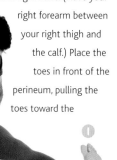

body with your right hand while your left hand pushes the heel forward to a vertical position. This is a strong position for many people. Those who aren't ready to fold forward can practice sitting erect. For many people, their yoga will include practice at remaining content while venturing only this far into the pose.

2 Set up the twist this pose requires by rotating the abdomen left. On an inhalation, stretch the right hand and shoulder forward to take hold of the inner left foot.

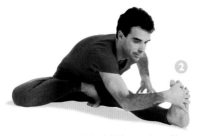

3 As you exhale, fold forward, working toward resting your head on the left shin and stretching the crown of the head toward the toes.

4 Bring your left hand forward to grasp the right wrist beyond the foot. If you are very flexible, rest your chin on your shin and gaze forward. This is the full Toe Stretching Head Beyond The Knee Pose.

5 Regardless of just where you arrive, work in the pose by drawing in the lower abdominal muscles (see Abdominal Lock, page 338) on each inhalation. This will give a lifting sensation to enable the chest to move farther forward on each exhalation—feel as if you are creeping your floating ribs farther along your thigh toward your knee.

6 Inhale to come up. Return to Seated Staff Posture, then repeat on the other side.

INFORMATION

GAZE Front big toe.

BUILD-UP POSES Head Beyond the Knee Pose, Cobbler's Pose, Toe Stretching Forward Bend.

COUNTER POSES Seated Staff Posture and Boat Pose, both while stretching out the toes and extending fully through the knee. East Stretch Posture.

LIGHTEN a) Do not go to the final stage. **b)** Hold the thigh, calf, or ankle of the straight leg if you can't reach the foot, or loop a soft belt around the ball of the foot.

EFFECT Calming.

Lotus Posture

Padmasana This is the most classic of yoga postures and, by reducing circulation (and therefore distracting sensations) to the legs, one of the best for meditation and pranayama. The Buddha is often pictured sitting in Lotus Posture.

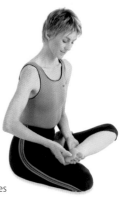

1 Practice Lotus Posture after working with the preparatory positions detailed with Cow Posture (page 140) and Half Bound Lotus Forward Bend (page 146).

2 Sit in Seated Staff Posture (page 140). Bend the right knee and hold the right foot with both hands. From this raised foot position, rather than just lowering the right heel to the left

thigh, get a sense of rolling the ball of the thighbone in the hip joint so the right knee comes to point forward rather than out to the right, and the fronts of the hipbones move closer together. Bring the right foot as far as possible up the left thigh, heel close to the navel. This is sometimes called Half Lotus Pose. Place your hands on your shin and front thigh just near the knee and squeeze them together, putting a beneficial force through your knee.

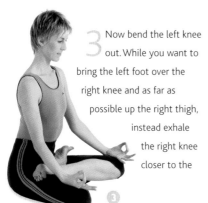

3 Now bend the left knee out. While you want to bring the left foot over the right knee and as far as possible up the right thigh, instead exhale the right knee closer to the floor so that the left ankle can slip up over it and slide along the thigh. Ⓐ The soles of both feet should be facing upward. Ⓑ If you experience pain in the knees, work with the build up poses instead. As Lotus Posture creates a small curve in the lower back, change whichever leg bends first each time you practice it.

CAUTION

According to the *Hatha Yoga Pradipika*, "Lotus Posture cures all diseases." However, it requires supple knees and hips, and many people in the West find it a very advanced posture, rather than a beginner's pose. Many yoga practitioners have found it requires a decade or more of dedicated yoga practice to be able to assume Lotus Posture safely. Never, ever force the legs into this posture, since this may seriously damage the knees. With consistent practice—a key to success in yoga—the hips and knees will gradually become flexible enough to sit comfortably.

INFORMATION

GAZE Straight ahead with a level gaze, or eyes closed.

BUILD-UP POSES Perfect Pose, Cobbler's Pose, Half Lotus Pose preparations, Cow Posture, Half Bound Lotus Forward Bend, Sage Pose B, Bound Sage Twist.

COUNTER POSES Hero Pose, Seated Staff Posture.

LIGHTEN a) Bring the left foot under the right leg, rather than above it. **b)** A simple cross-legged position is good for sitting practices.

EFFECT Calming, meditative.

Bound Lotus Posture

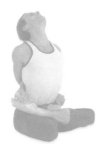

Baddha Padmasana In this continuation of Lotus Posture (page 152), the hands are crossed behind the back to catch the feet. This stretches the shoulders back strongly, opens the chest, and lessens the curvature of the upper spine. The forward-bending version also assists digestion.

1 Sit in Lotus Posture(page 152) with your right leg folded before your left. When you assume the pose, have your knees as close together as possible and the heels high up on the thighs, so the feet overhang slightly.

2 Take the left hand behind the back. Lean forward to grasp the big left toe. Twist the torso to the left and use your right hand to pull your left wrist if necessary.

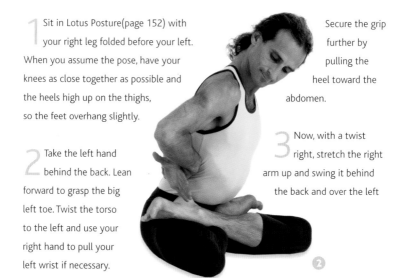

Secure the grip further by pulling the heel toward the abdomen.

3 Now, with a twist right, stretch the right arm up and swing it behind the back and over the left

2

arm so that the elbows are close together. Reach for the right foot with the right hand. In the beginning, it helps to lean forward slightly as you are securing the grip of the hand on the left foot. Sit up straight, drawing the abdomen in, pulling the shoulders back and lifting the chest as you turn the face skyward.

4 A new posture is created by leaning forward, folding the torso over the heels to bring the chin to the floor with the hands still binding. This is called Yoga Seal Position, a more difficult version of the pose outlined with Perfect Pose

(page 112). Come up on an inhalation, release the hands, then straighten the legs and repeat on the other side.

INFORMATION

GAZE Tip of nose.

BUILD-UP POSES Lotus Posture, Half Bound Lotus Twist.

COUNTER POSE Hero Pose.

LIGHTEN a) Grasp two belts looped around the feet. **b)** Rather than holding the feet, interlock the fingers behind the back or cup both elbows with the opposite hand.

EFFECT Calming.

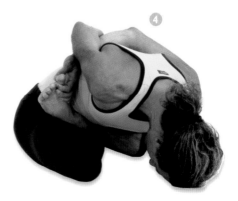

Fetus in the Womb Posture

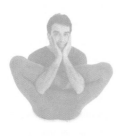

Garbha Pindasana In this continuation of Lotus Posture (page 152), the hands are inserted between the thighs and the calves. In addition to the usual benefits of Lotus Posture, this posture tones the abdominal organs. Before attempting it, it is essential to first master Lotus Posture.

1 Sit in Lotus Posture (page 152), right leg folded in first. Ensure your knees are close together and your heels high up on the thighs.

2 Insert the right hand between the right thigh and the right calf. (Unless you have very slender legs— and a very advanced Lotus Posture—there isn't much space there, so it might help to lubricate the forearms with warm water before attempting to thread them through.) Gently push the arm through until you can bend the elbow.

3 Now insert the left hand between the left thigh and the left calf until you can

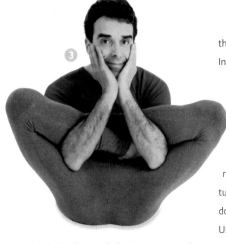

the sitting bones for several long breaths. Inhale, release the arms, then straighten the legs and repeat on the opposite side.

4 From Fetus In The Womb Posture, advanced practitioners of Ashtanga Vinyasa yoga (page 385) rock back and forth on their backs, turning round a little each time as they do so until they've done a complete circle. Use a cushioned surface. The momentum of the last forward roll brings them up into Rooster Posture, where the arms support the entire body weight.

bend the elbow. Pull the knees toward the chest, bend both elbows to bring the hands on either side of the face, if possible bringing the fingers to the ears. Balance on

INFORMATION

GAZE Tip of nose.

BUILD-UP POSE Lotus Posture.

COUNTER POSES Hero Pose, East Stretch Posture.

LIGHTEN a) Instead of threading them through, wrap the arms around the legs, bringing the knees to the chest.

EFFECT Calming.

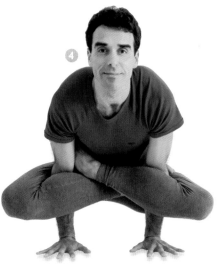

Plank Pose

Kumbhakasana In this pose, the body
is held strong and straight like a plank.
Similar to a push up, this pose strengthens
the arms and wrists and tones the
abdominal muscles. The upper back is
expanded fully, increasing oxygenation
of the muscle tissue and the release of
tension held between the shoulder blades.

1 Kneel on the floor with the hands
shoulder width apart. Have your
hands in front of the shoulders and lean
more weight forward onto them. Push
strongly through the palms of the hands
as if you are lengthening your arms. Press
the vertebrae between the shoulder blades
up toward the ceiling, so that the skin
between the shoulder blades widens and
the upper back broadens. Keep the back of
the neck long, face looking down and

chin tucked in slightly toward the throat.
Fully involve your abdominal muscles by
drawing them back toward the spine.
This is Kneeling Plank Pose.

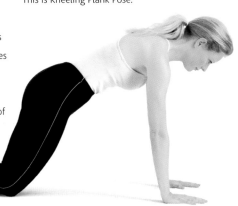

GAZE Tip of nose.

BUILD-UP POSES Downward Facing Dog Pose, Four Limbed Staff Pose.

COUNTER POSES Locust Pose, Supported Bridge Pose, Wrist Releases.

LIGHTEN a) Stay at the first stage, Kneeling Plank Pose. **b)** Hold for a short time.

EFFECT Strengthening.

abdominal muscles to firm them. If your buttocks lift in a mountain shape, check that your shoulders are correctly positioned. Bring your weight forward so your shoulders line up over your wrists—you might need to walk your hands forward.

3 Now round up the upper back to broaden the back and spread the shoulder blades apart. Squeeze the buttocks together and draw the pubic abdomen gently in toward the spine. Condense from the pubic bone to the lower ribs. Lengthen the tailbone toward the heels. Press the palms evenly to the floor. Hold for five breaths. From Plank Pose, you may lower into Four Limbed Staff Pose (page 160), or lift up to Downward Facing Dog Pose (page 162).

2 Tuck your toes under and lift the knees up. Bring your hips into line so that everything from the back of the head through the sacrum to the back of the heels is on one plane. Take care not to sink the hips too low—if you are collapsing into a valley, reestablish the workings of your

Four Limbed Staff Pose

Chaturanga Dandasana In this strengthening posture, often referred to as Crocodile Pose, the weight of the body rests on the hands and feet. It works the arms, wrists, and shoulders and tones the abdomen. It is one of the postures of some of the Sun Salutation (page 42) sequences.

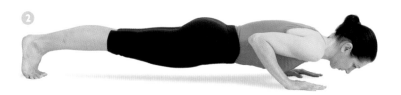

1 Lie on the floor on your stomach. Bend the elbows and place the hands flat on the floor underneath the shoulders, with the fingers pointing forward. Tuck the toes under, with the feet about 10 inches (25 centimeters) apart.

2 Firm the abdominal muscles and lift the whole body off the floor, so that the weight is entirely on the hands and toes, with the chest between the thumbs. Keep the whole body very straight. Draw your abdomen in toward your core so that as you lift up, you don't leave your belly behind! This will prevent sagging in the posture. Do not lift the buttocks high. Send a line of energy backward through the heels and shoot it forward through the crown of the head. Hug the elbows close to the body. Stay for ten breaths or more.

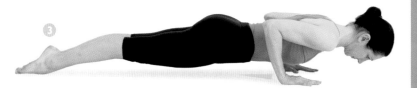

3 An alternative is to exhale and roll forward over the toes, so that your weight is supported only by the top of the feet and the hands. This puts extra pressure on the shoulders and arms. From this position, you can then roll back over the toes to the starting position or, as in Sun Salutation B sequence (page 42), straighten the elbows and continue on to Upward Facing Dog Pose (page 244).

4 To come into Four Limbed Staff Pose from Plank Pose (page 158), firm your abdomen and move your shoulders forward of your fingertips while at the same time bending the elbows to right angles. To avoid the feeling of crash landing, the chest needs to move forward and your nose will come close to the floor about one foot (30 centimeters) in front of the fingertips.

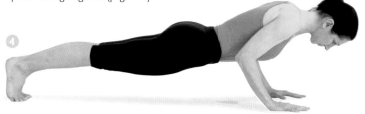

INFORMATION

GAZE Tip of nose.

BUILD-UP POSE Plank Pose.

COUNTER POSES Upward Facing Dog Pose, Wrist Releases.

LIGHTEN a) Do not roll forward to the last stage. **b)** Bend the knees and let them touch the floor to lighten the weight on the hands. **c)** Let the weight of the body rest on the floor, simply pressing the hands down.

EFFECT Energizing.

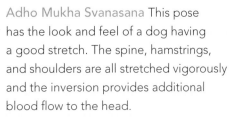

Downward Facing Dog Pose

Adho Mukha Svanasana This pose has the look and feel of a dog having a good stretch. The spine, hamstrings, and shoulders are all stretched vigorously and the inversion provides additional blood flow to the head.

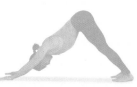

1 Stand in Mountain Pose (page 46). Inhale as you raise the arms over the head. Exhale and fold forward from the hips into Deep Forward Fold (page 68), hands beside the feet. Inhale and look forward, raising the chest away from the thighs. On an exhalation, step the right foot and then the left foot back (or jump them lightly back together). Have the feet and hands at least 3 feet (90 centimeters) apart.

2 Place your feet hip width apart with the legs straight and strong. Ensure your middle fingers point forward and that you are not taking the weight only on the little finger side of the hands. Press the palms evenly into the floor and move your chest closer toward your thighs as you press the sitting bones of the buttocks upward, lengthening the spine. Move your hips back and up, away from the wrists.

3 Once you have reached maximum upward extension of the spine, focus on opening the backs of the legs. Press down through the heels and fully straighten the knees, without locking them. If the soles

INFORMATION

GAZE Navel.

BUILD-UP POSES Deep Forward Fold, Cow Posture (shoulders), Plank Pose, Wide Leg Forward Bend (wrists).

COUNTER POSES Mountain Pose, Wrist Releases, Standing

Half Bow Balance

LIGHTEN a) Bend the knees in toward the chest. **b)** Take knees to the floor, buttocks high in the air, and stretch arms forward.

EFFECT Strengthening, invigorating.

of the feet come fully to the floor, step your feet farther back to give yourself more of a challenge.

4 Rotate your shoulders externally so that the upper arms move away from the ears. Let the crown of the head come closer to the floor so that the back of the neck is long. Tuck your chin in and look toward the navel.

5 Stay here for ten to thirty breaths, breathing smoothly and deeply to enliven the whole body. Release on an inhalation, by looking forward as you step or jump the feet forward between the hands. Exhale into Deep Forward Fold, head toward the knees, then inhale and raise the arms and upper body back up to stand in Mountain Pose.

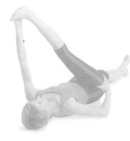

Reclining Hand to Toe Sequence

Supta Padangusthasana This posture stretches the hamstring muscles, limbers the legs and hip joints, and releases the lower back. As the back is kept fairly steady, it reduces the risk of back strain that may accompany a seated or standing forward bend.

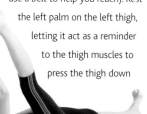

1 Lie on your back with the feet together. Bring the right leg straight up without bending the knee. Reach upward with the right hand and catch the big toe with the index and the middle fingers (or use a belt to help you reach). Rest the left palm on the left thigh, letting it act as a reminder to the thigh muscles to press the thigh down and make sure that it does not turn out. Keep the left foot active, either by pointing the toes or strongly flexing the ankle to press the heel away. A great way to keep this leg active is to lie perpendicular to the wall and press the heel into it.

2 After one to two minutes, raise the head and use your abdominal muscles to lift the chest toward the right

knee. At the same time bring the right leg closer to the torso so as to bring the head to the right shin. Hold for five breaths.

3 Lower the back of the head to the floor and externally rotate the right leg so the toes point out to the side. As you keep the hips even, lower the leg to the right side. At a certain point your left leg may lose its anchoring and you may feel that you will tip over. If so, come back

up and reestablish a strong anchor by pressing the left thigh down and the heel of the left foot away. Come slowly back to your maximum. Turn the head to the left. Hold for five to ten slow breaths.

4 Bring the right leg back up to center and catch the inside of the right foot with the left hand. Internally rotate the whole leg so the toes turn in. Hook your right thumb in the groove where the thigh and torso meet. Press into the groove to keep the right side of the waist long. Take the right leg across the body to the left, keeping the right side of the sacrum anchored to the floor. Turn the head to look to the right. Hold for five to ten breaths. Repeat on the other side.

INFORMATION

GAZE Big toe/side.

BUILD-UP POSES Seated Forward Bends.

COUNTER POSE Supported Bridge Pose.

LIGHTEN a) Hold the ankle instead of the big toe. **b)** Grasp a belt looped around the ball of the raised foot.

EFFECT Restful.

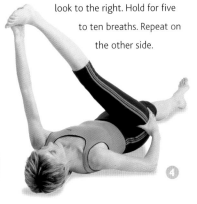

Monkey God Posture

Hanumanasana This challenging yet graceful posture, which resembles the splits performed by ballet dancers and gymnasts, strongly stretches the muscles of the front and back thighs. It is named after Hanuman, the monkey god. It refers to the fantastic leaps this popular deity took in service to his master Rama.

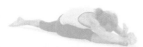

1 Kneel on the floor and step the right leg to the front. Bring the hands to the floor on either side of the body. Straighten the right leg and slide the right heel forward until the calf muscles touch the floor.

2 At the same time, slide the left knee and foot back, with the toes pointing straight back, until the front of the left thigh touches the floor. Press the legs and hips down. Adjust the hips. Bring the left hip forward so the hips are squared off to the front.

Ensure the front leg points straight ahead. Have the kneecap facing straight up so the leg is not turned out to the side.

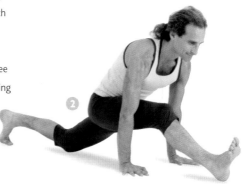

INFORMATION

GAZE Tip of nose.

BUILD-UP POSES Lunges, Head Beyond the Knee Pose, Single Leg Forward Bend, Single Leg Swan Balance, Reclining Half Hero Pose, Frog Pose, Crescent Moon Pose.

COUNTER POSES Hero Pose, Corpse Pose.

LIGHTEN a) Keep hands on the floor. **b)** Use blocks to support under the perineum or the hands. **c)** Do not go to the forward bending position.

EFFECT Calming.

3 Once the legs are straight, sit on the floor and bring the hands together in a prayer position in front of the chest or else raise to prayer position with arms straight up in the air. Stay in this position for ten breaths or more. Then fold forward on an exhalation, and hold the left wrist with the right hand beyond the foot, resting the head on the right shin.

4 To come out of the posture, place the hands back down on either side of the body and lift the body up. After this strong release, take care to support with the hands as you bring your legs closer together. Alternate the legs to repeat on the other side, holding for the same length of time. Often people find one side easier. In this case, hold the stiffer side for longer.

Seated Leg Behind the Head Posture

Eka Pada Sirsasana This posture works into the hips and stimulates blood flow to the pelvic and abdominal regions. This extreme forward bend puts a lot of pressure on the lower back and neck and should be approached with caution.

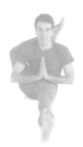

1 Sit in Seated Staff Posture (page 104). Draw the right knee up and catch the right foot with the left hand. Place the right hand on the floor beside the right hip, with the arm inside the right knee.

2 Bring the right knee back and straighten the right leg, gradually bringing the right hand back and the knee as far behind the right shoulder as possible. The right knee must be behind the shoulder to continue to the next step.

3 Exhale, catch the calf with the right hand, pressing the whole leg farther back, and with the help of both hands, lift the right foot

❶

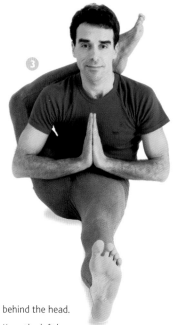

INFORMATION

GAZE Tip of nose.

BUILD-UP POSES Tortoise Posture and Sleeping Tortoise Posture, One Legged Cobra Pose.

COUNTER POSES Corpse Pose, East Stretch Posture, Camel Posture.

LIGHTEN a) Do not bring the foot behind the head. **b)** Support the chin with both hands to help straighten the neck in the final upright position. **c)** Do not go to the final (reclining) stage.

EFFECT Calming.

behind the head.
Keep the left leg
straight, with the toes pointing up.
Straighten the back and neck as much as
possible and lift the chin to look forward.
Bring the hands together in prayer position
in front of the chest.

4 Gradually lie back, keeping the left foot on the floor. This posture is called Bhairava Pose, named after Bhairava, an aspect of the Hindu god Shiva. Inhale, rock back to sitting, release the right leg and straighten it out. Repeat on the other side.

Tortoise and Sleeping Tortoise Postures

Supta Kurma Asana In these postures, the back resembles the shell of a tortoise. The postures stretch the lower back, tone the abdominal organs, open the hips, and calm the nervous system.

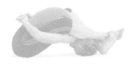

1 Sit in Seated Staff Posture (page 104). Bend the knees slightly, rolling the legs outward, and place the feet about 2 feet (60 centimeters) apart. Bend forward from the hips and roll slightly to one side, then the other, to slide the arms one by one underneath the knees. Rock from side to side again to take the shoulders as close to the knees as possible. Extend the arms out to the side.

2 Keep bending forward and look straight ahead. Slide the feet away to bring the chin and the shoulders to the floor. Lengthen the front of the body and bring the chest

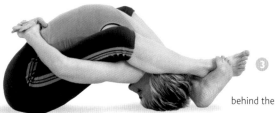

toward the floor. Straighten the legs and roll them in so that the knees are pointing up. Lift the feet off the floor, so the backs of the knees press the shoulders down. Broaden the chest. This is Tortoise Posture. Stay for ten breaths or more.

3 Internally rotate the shoulders and bend the elbows to bring the arms back near the hips. Rock a little from side to side if necessary. Take the hands behind the lumbar region of the spine and clasp them firmly. Move the feet one by one toward the center and, above the head, cross the legs at the ankles. This is Sleeping Tortoise Posture. Stay for ten breaths or more. Then change the position of the feet and repeat the posture for the same length of time on the other side.

4 Inhale, bend the knees a little, wiggle the shoulders out from underneath the knees, and then sit up.

INFORMATION

GAZE Third eye.

BUILD-UP POSES Wide Leg Forward Bend, Seated Angle Posture, Reclining Hand to Toe Sequence Cycle, Seated Leg Behind the Head Posture.

COUNTER POSES East Stretch Posture, Upward Facing Dog Pose, Downward Facing Dog Pose.

LIGHTEN a) Rest the forehead, rather than the chin, on the floor in Tortoise Posture. **b)** Do not straighten the legs in Tortoise Posture. **c)** Do not cross the ankles in Sleeping Tortoise Posture. **d)** Grasp a belt between the hands in Sleeping Tortoise Posture.

EFFECT Calming.

Yogic Sleep Pose

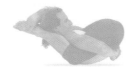

Yoga Nidrasana This is one of the strongest forward bends. Once mastered, it is a very relaxing posture and contributes to the health of the whole body. This forward bend improves blood flow to the abdominal region and the digestive system in particular.

1 Prepare your body with a sequence of forward bends. A further preparation is to lie on your back, hold one foot with both hands, and bring it up to the forehead while you press the knee down toward the floor. After practicing on both sides, do both feet together.

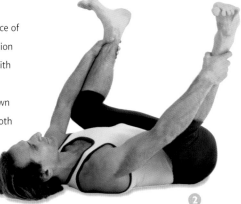

2

2 Lie on your back. Bend both knees and take hold of the ankles or, if possible, the heels. Start to pull the knees toward the floor near your armpits, while your feet move beyond the level of the head. Let your lower back lift off the floor to deepen the forward bend. Take your time and work with a long steady exhalation.

3 When ready, lift your head off the floor and move your hands to your outer heels. Pull your shoulders through one at a time, so the knees move up over the shoulders. Rock a little from one side to the other if necessary.

4 Cross the ankles one at a time behind the head. With legs locked in place, move your shoulders up so that they are well above the knees and work on opening the chest. Extend the arms away from the torso, and internally rotating from the shoulder, bring the hands back one by one and clasp them behind the back.

INFORMATION

GAZE Upward.

BUILD-UP POSES Seated Leg Behind the Head Posture, Tortoise Posture.

COUNTER POSES East Stretch Posture, Downward Facing Dog Pose, Upward Facing Dog Pose, Camel Posture.

LIGHTEN Practice one leg at a time.

EFFECT Calming.

Lift the chest back and rest the head back on the "pillow" formed by your feet. Stay in this position for ten breaths or more.

5 Release the hands and repeat with the legs crossed the opposite way.

Twists & Abdominal Toners

Your center of gravity lies in the abdomen. At this core of the body is the workhouse for the all-important abdominal organs. Twists bring fresh, oxygen-rich blood to the organs and the bowel, nourishing them. Together with the massaging effect of the twisting action, they promote healthy functioning, digestion, and elimination. Toning the abdominal muscles is vital for good posture and protection from lower back pain.

Twisting around gives you a chance to see things from a new perspective. Twists release a lot of tension from the small muscles around the spine. They are great balancers.

When you are restless and agitated, twists tend to settle you down. They give you a lift when you feel tired and lethargic. The next time you get wound up by life, spiral yourself into a long twist, then, as your body uncoils, feel your mind unwind.

Double Leg Raises

Urdhva Prasarita Padasana This pose
is a fantastic tummy toner! It strengthens
the muscles of the lower back and
abdomen. There are many possible
variations, so do experiment to find which
ones challenge you most and which make
the pose more achievable.

1 Lie flat on your back, legs extended, arms along the floor overhead,
and backs of the hands pressing to the floor. As you inhale, stretch
the arms over the head to reach the floor behind you and lift the legs
toward the ceiling. Draw the lower abdomen in toward the spine as you
exhale and lower the legs back to the floor. Repeat five to ten more
times. The more slowly and controlled you can work, the better. Don't
hold the breath, but keep it flowing steadily so your movement can be
perfectly timed to the breath.

2 You may like to lower the legs in stages, holding for several breaths each when they are at 60° and 30°, then again when the heels are 2 inches (5 centimeters) from the floor. The abdominal muscles are working at their maximum here, so persevere with this last stage. Breathe deeply and evenly. Keep the shoulders relaxed.

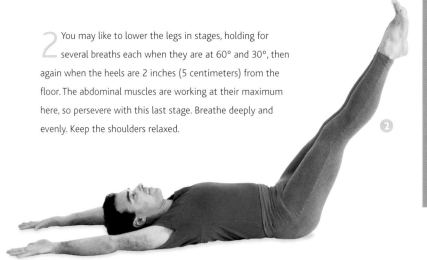

INFORMATION

GAZE Tip of nose.

BUILD-UP POSES Boat Pose, Plank Pose, Revolved Abdomen Pose, Extended Leg Fish Pose.

COUNTER POSES Reclining Bound Angle Pose, Corpse Pose.

LIGHTEN a) Bend the knees. **b)** Bend the knees and have your feet on the floor behind the buttocks. **c)** Hold the knees with your hands. As you exhale, bend the elbows and draw the knees to the chest. On each inhalation, open the arms above the head and stretch the feet toward the ceiling. **d)** Release the legs and arms to the floor on the exhalation.

EFFECT Strengthening.

All these variations can be done instead with the hands under the sacrum or palms to floor by the hips.

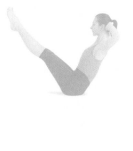

Boat Pose

Navasana This pose is one of the best for strengthening and toning the abdominal organs. It also works the muscles of the lower back. It is very challenging at first, but consistent practice will give benefits sooner rather than later.

1 Sit in Seated Staff Posture (page 104) with the hands beside the hips on the floor. On an exhalation, lean the body back slightly as you bend the knees and lift the legs off the floor. Bend the knees so your shins are parallel to the floor. Hold behind your thighs with your hands. Draw in the lower back so it is more of a concave shape. Lift the heart center. Stretch the arms forward so the palms are facing each other. Pull the shoulders back and lift the chest forward (toward the knees), opening the heart as you extend through the fingers. Breathe here for five to eight breaths. Then rest and repeat or progress to Stage 2.

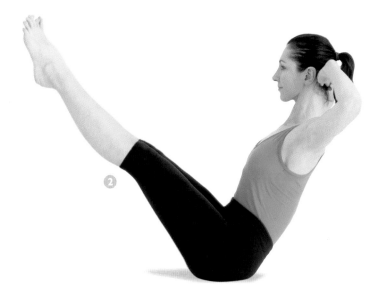

INFORMATION

GAZE Toes.

BUILD-UP POSES Chair Pose, Double Leg Raises, Extended Leg Fish Pose.

COUNTER POSES Corpse Pose, East Stretch Posture.

LIGHTEN a) At the first stage, rest the toes lightly on the floor. **b)** Keep the knees bent. **c)** Hold for a short time.

EFFECT Strengthening.

2 To practice the full Boat Pose from a knees-bent position, slowly straighten the legs upward until they are fully extended. Have the feet higher than the head. With the abdominal muscles working strongly, focus on keeping the legs extended and the upper body lifting so the back doesn't round out. If you are very strong, interlace the fingers behind the head, keeping elbows wide, taking care not to sag into the lower back or collapse the chest toward the belly. After five to eight breaths, release on an exhalation.

Revolved Easy Pose

Parivrtta Sukhasana Happiness is felt in the heart center. In this pose, the heart rests gently down into the supportive foundation of the pelvis. Enjoy the sensation of fullness this pose offers.

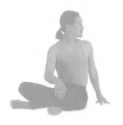

1 Cross your legs and slide your heels well apart so that each heel rests near or under the knee above it. (Your shin bones will be more or less parallel.) Place your fingertips on the floor directly behind your buttocks, fingers pointing away from you.

2 Press both sitting bones evenly into the floor and gently draw the lower spine inward and upward. Breathe all the way down into the perineum as you lengthen upward through the spine and the sides of the body. Soften the diaphragm at the edge of the lower ribs, allowing the lungs to release down to caress the abdomen.

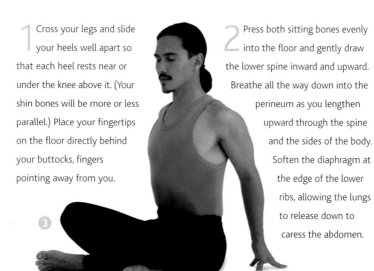

4 Raise both arms toward the ceiling. Lengthen upward from hips to armpits, then from the armpits all the way out through to the fingertips. Keeping the upper body as long and spacious as possible, exhale and turn the chest toward the left. For a moment observe which muscles are helping you twist.

5 Placing the right hand on the outer left knee and your left hand to the floor by your side and a little back, use them to lever you deeply into the twist. Keep the chin drawn in slightly and both shoulders level. Stay here for ten breaths, gently drawing the pubic abdomen in toward the spine and expanding the heart and chest as you inhale, then twisting more as you exhale.

3 Inhale deeply across the base of the chest so it widens. Breathe into the heart. Soften the upper chest. Gently draw the chin toward the throat. Notice how far down the torso your breath is carrying. Can it fill the basin of the pelvis?

6 Release on an inhalation and sit for a moment in the center, eyes closed, feeling the effects of having done just one side. Repeat on the other side.

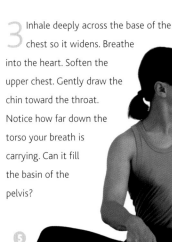

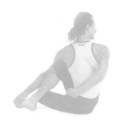

Seated Half Spinal Twist

Ardha Matsyendrasana The pressure of thigh against abdomen massages the internal organs and promotes their healthy functioning.

1 From Seated Staff Posture (page 104), bend both knees and place the feet on the floor. Bend the left knee and take the foot back toward the the right buttock. Have the heel directly in front of the right sitting bone.

2 Take the right leg up and over the left thigh so the foot comes near the left knee. Press both sitting bones down toward the floor. Draw the lower back slightly in and up, releasing the spine up toward the crown of the head. While the right fingertips press to the floor, inhale and stretch the left arm upward, extending through the fingers.

3 Exhale and turn the abdomen and chest toward the right. Without losing the length in the torso,

bring your left elbow to the outer right thigh. Push against the thigh while resisting with it to assist in twisting to the right.

reach the hand to the front of the right foot. Wrap your right hand around the back of your body. Gaze over your right shoulder.

4 Move the left elbow to the outside of the right knee, without shortening the left side of the waist. Bring the left armpit as close to the knee as possible, maintaining the extension of the spine. Straighten the left arm and

5 Breathe here, gently squeezing the lower abdomen in toward the spine on the exhalation and lifting the chest and lengthening the spine on the exhalation to deepen the twist.

6 Release on an inhalation, letting go of the hands and returning the chest to the center. Unfold the legs, rest in Seated Staff Posture, and repeat on the other side.

INFORMATION

FOCUS Over the back shoulder.

COUNTER POSES East Stretch Posture, Double Leg Forward Stretch.

BUILD-UP POSES Revolved Easy Pose, Bound Sage Pose.

LIGHTEN a) Hug the front knee with the opposite arm while pressing the torso to thigh. **b)** If you are unable to clasp the hands, allow the back hand to rest on the floor and have the front elbow bent to 90°, fingers pointing toward the sky. **c)** An intermediate option is to put the right arm through the "window" under the knee to grasp the left hand.

EFFECT Balancing—both invigorating and calming.

Sage Twist

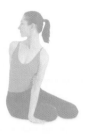

Bharadvajasana This simple twist is very effective for releasing tension in the neck, shoulders, and spine. When we twist to both sides, we can find our center. This twist is an opportunity to turn our attention inward to discover the wisdom we have deep within our own bodies.

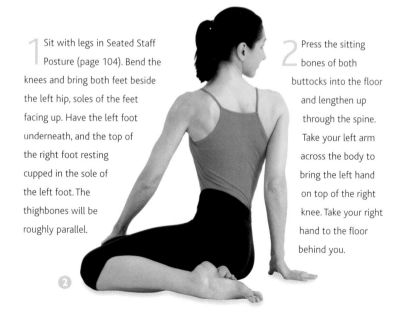

1 Sit with legs in Seated Staff Posture (page 104). Bend the knees and bring both feet beside the left hip, soles of the feet facing up. Have the left foot underneath, and the top of the right foot resting cupped in the sole of the left foot. The thighbones will be roughly parallel.

2 Press the sitting bones of both buttocks into the floor and lengthen up through the spine. Take your left arm across the body to bring the left hand on top of the right knee. Take your right hand to the floor behind you.

3 Inhale and float the torso longer. Exhale, and keeping the length in the spine, spiral into a deep upward moving twist from the lower left abdomen to the right shoulder.

4 Inhale and reestablish the length through the torso. Lean forward and, with left inner wrist turned out, slide the fingers under the right knee. Now take the right arm behind the waist and clasp the upper left arm with the right hand. It helps to lean farther forward to grip. Once you have the grip, bring the spine more to vertical once again. Tuck your chin in and turn the head to gaze over the right shoulder.

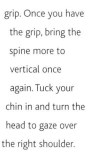

INFORMATION

GAZE To side.

BUILD-UP POSE Revolved Easy Pose, Seated Half Spinal Twist.

COUNTER POSES East Stretch Posture, Double Leg Forward Stretch, Cross Legged Forward Stretch, Extended Child Pose, Downward Facing Dog Pose.

LIGHTEN a) Stay at the first stage. **b)** Place a cushion under your left buttock. **c)** Keep the left hand on the floor instead of behind the waist.

EFFECT Centering.

5 Breathe here for five to ten breaths, elongating the spine on each inhalation and gently squeezing farther into the twist on each exhalation. Press the back of the wrist away from your torso and move your right shoulder farther back to deepen the twist. Anchor more through the left sitting bone.

6 Release the arms as you inhale, stretch the legs out, and repeat on the other side.

Twisting Forward Stretches

Parivrtta Paschimottanasana and
Utthita Parivrtta Paschimottanasana
In these forward bends the whole spine
and backs of the legs are stretched, the
abdominal organs are contracted
strongly, and the kidneys are squeezed,
rejuvenating the blood system of the body.

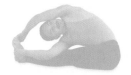

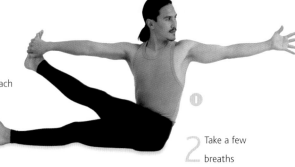

1 From Seated Staff
Posture (page 104), reach
forward and grasp the
outer left foot with
the right hand (bend
the knee if necessary).
Inhale and raise the left leg off the floor as
you lift the trunk of the body upright. Now
twist the whole upper body toward the
left, extending the left arm out at shoulder
height behind the body. Have the palm
facing outward and turn the head to gaze
over the left shoulder. This is a twisting
forward stretch.

2 Take a few
breaths
here, lifting the leg and the spine upward
on each inhalation, and deepening into the
twist from the pubic abdomen on every
exhalation. Release to the front, on an
exhalation, lower the raised leg, and
extend both arms over your head. Return
to Seated Staff Posture and repeat on the
other side.

3 For Revolved Stretch on the West Side of the Body, first sit in Seated Staff Posture. Inhale as you raise the arms above the head. Cross the arms at the wrists and exhale as you extend the upper body forward and catch hold of the feet with the hands. The right hand holds the left foot and the left hand holds the right foot. Have your left wrist above the right.

4 Take a few breaths to warm up to this forward bending position. Then, lift your left elbow and armpit higher and start to turn your abdomen and chest up toward the sky. Turn your face to look up under your upper left arm.

5 Lengthen the heels away even as your hands pull back on the feet to give you more twist. On each exhalation, draw the pubic abdomen in toward the spine and revolve to the right more deeply. After five to ten breaths here, repeat on the other side.

INFORMATION

GAZE To back thumb or all the way around to the side.

BUILD-UP POSES Double Leg Forward Stretch, Revolved Abdomen Pose, Revolved Chair Pose.

COUNTER POSES Reclining Bound Angle Pose, Corpse Pose, East Stretch Posture.

LIGHTEN a) Have knee(s) bent **b)** First stage—keep hand of raised leg on floor behind buttock. **c)** Loop a belt around the raised foot. **d)** Second stage—keep both hands on opposite knees.

EFFECT Centering.

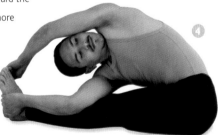

Seated Gate Pose

Vira Parighasana The linear movements we repeat each day tend to restrict the fullness of who we are, but the unusual shape of this pose invites us to open our view. It expands the intercostal muscles to allow the breath to move more freely into the lungs.

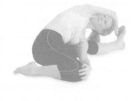

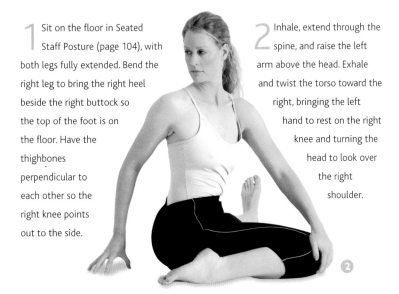

1 Sit on the floor in Seated Staff Posture (page 104), with both legs fully extended. Bend the right leg to bring the right heel beside the right buttock so the top of the foot is on the floor. Have the thighbones perpendicular to each other so the right knee points out to the side.

2 Inhale, extend through the spine, and raise the left arm above the head. Exhale and twist the torso toward the right, bringing the left hand to rest on the right knee and turning the head to look over the right shoulder.

2

3 Bend the left knee up so the heel is on the floor. Inhale and stretch the spine upward. As you exhale, keeping the belly and chest rotated toward the right, bring the left shoulder down to the inside of the left knee.

4 Inhale as you stretch the right arm upward and over the head to grasp hold of the big toe of the extended left foot. Grasp hold of the extended left foot. Pull back on your left foot to curve your right side ribs upward. The feeling will be one of spreading the ribs apart and distributing the side bend more evenly through the spine. Grip your right knee and bend the left elbow. Ease the torso deeper into the twist. Turn the head to gaze up under the upper right arm. Breathe here for as long as you are enjoying the twist.

5 Release as you inhale, lifting the torso up as you raise the arms and turn the chest to face forward. On the exhalation, lower the arms beside the hips. Repeat on the other side.

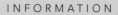

INFORMATION

GAZE Infinity.

BUILD-UP POSES Gate Pose, Bound Sage Pose, Revolved Chair Pose, Twisting Forward Stretches.

COUNTER POSES Child Pose, East Stretch Posture, Reclining Angle Pose.

LIGHTEN a) Bend the knee of the extended leg upward, bringing the foot closer. **b)** Stretch the top hand away overhead, rather than grasping your front foot.

EFFECT Releasing.

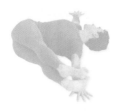

Revolved Abdomen Pose

Jathara Parivartanasana This supported spinal twist gently squeezes the abdominal organs, releasing stored toxins. The initial version can work wonders as a mobilizer and pain reliever for tight lower backs. The full pose is a strong abdominal toner.

3 Ⓐ

1 Lie flat on your back on the floor. Press the lower back into the floor and lengthen the spine. Open the arms to shoulder height, palms down on the floor.

2 Draw the chin in toward the chest, allowing the back of the neck to lengthen. Relax the shoulders away from the ears.

3 Ⓑ

3 Exhale and raise both knees toward the chest. Inhale and expand the breath in the chest. Ⓐ Exhale and drop both knees together toward the right. Keep both shoulders in contact with the floor and turn your head to the left. Ⓑ Inhale as you bring the knees back to the chest. Then exhale as you drop the knees to the left to practice on the other side.

4 After around five repetitions on each side, drop the knees to the right and hold for several long, luxurious breaths. On each inhalation, imagine the spine lengthening toward the crown of the head. On each exhalation, anchor down the back shoulder a little more. Experiment with the position of the knees.

Moving them closer to the armpit or farther away will change where you feel the stretch on the back.

5 Once you have warmed up in this easy version, practice the pose using straight legs if possible. First, swivel your hips to the right, so your toes point toward your left hand.

6 On an exhalation, lower your legs, toes aiming toward the fingertips. Inhale to come up, swivel the hips to the left, and repeat on the other side. Build to five repetitions on each side.

7 On the last repetition, legs to the left, hold the toes or side of the left foot with your hand and stretch both heels away as you revolve your abdomen to the right. Let the right side of your back press down to the floor as you gaze over the right hand. Stay for several breaths before repeating on the right side.

INFORMATION

GAZE To the back hand.

BUILD-UP POSES Double Leg Raises, Boat Pose, Revolved Easy Pose, Revolved Triangle Pose.

COUNTER POSES Locust Pose, East Stretch Posture.

LIGHTEN a) If your shoulder lifts up as your knees drop toward the floor, move that hand down toward the buttocks until both shoulders can come closer to the floor.
b) Leave the head looking upward if the neck is restricted.
c) Bend your knees rather than straightening them.

EFFECT Strengthening, centering.

Revolved Chair Pose

Parivrtta Utkatasana Squatting is a powerful innate body posture that puts us in touch with our connection to the earth. In this version, twisting the upper body gives the abdominal muscles a massage, while the legs are strengthened.

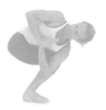

1 Stand in Mountain Pose (page 46) with the feet hip width apart. Inhale, extend the arms over the head and lengthen the spine. Exhale and fold forward with bent knees, bringing the chest toward the thighs, and hands to the floor. Inhale, press down into the soles and lift the arms and chest forward, away from the thighs. Keep lifting the chest, extending through the fingers until the spine and the arms are parallel to the floor.

2 Lift the sitting bones up toward the ceiling. Breathe smoothly and evenly as you establish a steady grounding through the heels. You will feel the thighs working hard. Lower the buttocks more toward the heels even as the arms and spine extend

INFORMATION

GAZE Sideways.

BUILD-UP POSES Deep Forward Fold, Chair Pose, Revolved Triangle Pose.

COUNTER POSES Mountain Pose, Tree Pose.

LIGHTEN a) Bend the knees less. **b)** Rest hands on the hip and knee of the side toward which you are turned.

EFFECT Invigorating.

upward more. Lower the hands to the heart and press the palms together in prayer position.

3 On an exhalation, turn the chest toward the right and lean forward to wedge the left elbow at the outer right knee. Press the elbow into the knee, while at the same time press the knee back to the elbow to twist deeper. Keep the thumbs at the breastbone and press the palms firmly together. Push the right knee forward to level it with the left. Feel a spiraling of the upper body from the sacrum upward. Turn the head to look over the right shoulder. Sit down more deeply into the buttocks. Move your body weight back slightly so that the knees are not too far forward of the ankles—this will engage the powerful muscles of the upper thighs more deeply. Stay here for five breaths.

4 Release as you inhale, allowing the arms to lift you back up to stand in Mountain Pose. Repeat on the other side.

Half Bound Lotus Twist

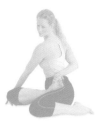

Bharadvajasana II This simple seated twist releases stiffness in the upper back and shoulders. While the twist might be less intense than in Sage Twist (page 184), the position of the legs makes it more of a challenge for those with tight hips.

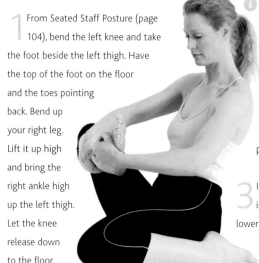

1 From Seated Staff Posture (page 104), bend the left knee and take the foot beside the left thigh. Have the top of the foot on the floor and the toes pointing back. Bend up your right leg. Lift it up high and bring the right ankle high up the left thigh. Let the knee release down to the floor.

2 Draw the abdominal muscles gently in toward the spine as you lengthen the tailbone down toward the floor. Lean backward slightly and press the sitting bones down.

3 Inhale, raise the right arm in the air. Moving from your lower abdomen, twist to your right. Lengthen as you rotate from your navel

right thigh. Have the inner wrist facing outward and press as much of the palm to the floor as possible. Spiraling upward from the lower abdomen, revolve the torso farther right and gaze over the left shoulder. Involve your eyeballs so they look as far around as possible. On each inhalation, lengthen up through the spine, and on each exhalation, twist more.

5 Release on an exhalation. Come back to Seated Staff Posture and repeat on the other side.

toward your right shoulder, then extend from the shoulder through to the fingertips of the right hand. Internally rotate the shoulder, bend the elbow, and bring the arm behind the waist to hold the toes of the right foot.

4 Still twisting, take the left hand across the body and wrap it under the

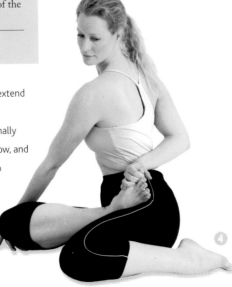

Spinal Twist in Half Lotus

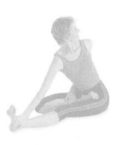

Ardha Padma Matsyendrasana This challenging twisting posture opens the hips, knees, and shoulders. Because of the pressure of the heel on the abdomen, it tones the abdominal organs and increases digestive power. Like all yoga postures, this is best practiced on an empty stomach.

1 Sit in Seated Staff Posture (page 104). Bend the right knee into Half Lotus Pose (page 152), drawing the heel close to the navel. If necessary, use the preparations outlined in Half Bound Lotus Forward Bend (page 146), and Cow Posture (page 140). Keep the kneecap of the left knee facing straight up, so the leg doesn't roll out to the side. Extend the left heel away.

2 Long arms really help in this twist! Rather than thinking of your arm starting at your shoulder, consider it as starting at your abdomen. Exhale and twist your abdomen to the left as you extend the left arm out to the side.

3 Internally rotate your left shoulder and take the arm around behind and grasp the inner right thigh. Still radiating from the navel, and moving your shoulder

INFORMATION

GAZE Back over the shoulder.

BUILD-UP POSES Half Bound Lotus Forward Bend, Half Bound Lotus Twist, Sage Pose B, Bound Sage Pose, Bound Sage Twist.

COUNTER POSES East Stretch Posture, Double Leg Forward Stretch.

LIGHTEN a) Do not put the left leg in Half Lotus Pose, but rest the foot on the floor near the inner thigh of the straight leg, as in Head Beyond the Knee Pose. **b)** Press your hand to the floor behind you, or grasp your thigh instead of the shin. **c)** Grasp a belt looped around the shin of the bent knee.

EFFECT Opening.

back, walk your fingers forward to grasp the right shin. Lean forward and use the other hand to help get the grasp.

4 Inhale, lift the chest, and straighten the back. Reach the right arm forward, then bring the hand down and catch the outer edge of the left foot. Turn the head to look back over the left shoulder. Twist deeply from the abdomen as you move your shoulder back and up to open your chest out to the side. Stay for ten breaths. Exhale, release the hands, sit up, come back to Seated Staff Posture, then repeat on the other side.

Bound Sage Pose

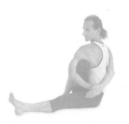

Marichyasana C This posture opens the hips, relieves backaches, and tones the abdominal organs. It also stretches the shoulders. It is a confining pose, as one part of your body is wedged against another, and it can sometimes be mentally confronting.

1 Sit in Seated Staff Posture (page 104). Bend the right knee and bring the right foot in front of the right sitting bone, with the sole of the foot pressing against the floor and the toes pointing straight forward. Leave 2–3 inches (5–8 centimeters) between the right foot and the inner left thigh. (An easier option in the beginning is to make the right foot slightly pigeon-toed, so the knee leans toward the center line of the body.) Place the right hand a few inches behind the right hip, fingers pointing backward. Place your left hand on your right outer knee. Exhale, draw in the abdomen and turn to

arrives near the left hip. Extend away with
the right arm, then wrap it around the
back and clasp the hands—if possible the
left hand holds the right wrist. Turn the
head the opposite way from the trunk so
you gaze forward over the left shoulder.
Do not lean back. Anchor down through
the sole of the right foot, particularly the
mound of the big toe.

the right. Take several breaths to deepen
the twist, using the support of your left
hand to lever your chest farther right.

2 When you are ready, bring the left
elbow over the right knee, armpit as
close to the outer knee as possible. Inhale,
lift the chest, and straighten the back,
lifting from the base of the spine, then
exhale and wrap the left
arm around the right
knee so the left hand

3 Deepen the twist by pressing the right
foot into the floor as if you want to
stand up, and moving the inner knee away
from the left armpit. Extend
through both elbows. Keep the
front (straight) leg energized
by stretching the heel
away. Stay for ten breaths.

4 Exhale, release the
hands, and
come to seated
Staff Posture. Then
repeat on the
other side.

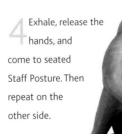

Bound Sage Twist

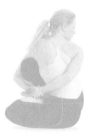

Marichyasana D This challenging twisting posture opens the hips, knees, and shoulders. Because of the pressure of the heel against the abdomen, it tones the abdominal organs and increases digestive power. Ensure you are well warmed up to lessen the risk of damaging your ankles and knees.

1 Sit in Seated Staff Posture (page 104). Bend the left knee into Half Lotus Pose (first practice the preparatory exercises on pages 140 and 146). Take plenty of time and several attempts so that you place the heel as close as possible to the navel. To avoid overstretching the ligaments of the outer foot, ensure more of the ankle is sitting on the top of the right thigh, rather than just the outer part of the foot.

2 Bend the right knee and bring the right foot in front of the right buttock bone. Have the toes pointing straight forward and the sole of the foot pressing well against the floor.

3 Take the left arm high in the air, lean back on the right hand, and breathe some length into your torso, particularly on the right side. Ⓐ As you exhale, turn to

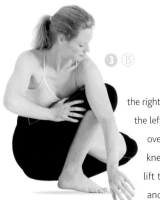

3 **(B)**

the right and bring
the left elbow
over the right
knee. Inhale,
lift the chest
and straighten
the back, then exhale, twisting deeply right
as you extend your armpit beyond the
right shin. Assist by pressing your thigh in
with the right hand. Rotate your shoulder
inward so the elbow points up. **(B)**

4 Wrap the left arm around the outer
right knee to bring the left hand back
near the left hip. Remaining well anchored
with the left upper arm pressing against
the right leg, bring the right arm up and
around the back to clasp the hands, left
hand holding right wrist. Turn the shoulders
and neck more to the right and look over
the right shoulder. Stay for ten breaths.

5 Exhale, release the hands and come
back to Seated Staff Posture. Then
repeat on the other side.

INFORMATION

GAZE Back over the shoulder.

BUILD-UP POSES Revolved Easy
Pose, Sage Pose B, Bound Sage
Pose, Half Bound Lotus Twist.

COUNTER POSE East Stretch
Posture. .

LIGHTEN a) If it is not possible
to bind the hands, catch the right
foot or the right hip with the left
hand and leave the right hand
on the floor behind the back.
b) Use a belt to link the hands
behind the back.

EFFECT Opening.

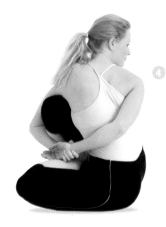

4

Noose Posture

Pasasana This challenging twisting posture, where the arms wrap rope-like around the legs, works the ankles and shoulders as well as giving the abdomen a strong twist. Until your heels happily come down to the floor, balance will be an added requirement of this posture.

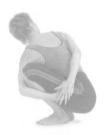

1 From Mountain Pose (page 46), squat down fully to sit on your heels with the knees together. Do not let your feet turn out, but keep the toes together. Rotate your abdomen fully to the right and put your right hand on the floor to balance. Deepen the twist by pressing the left hand to the outer right thigh, while also resisting with the thigh.

2 Continue releasing into this twist by pressing the left elbow against the left knee as you lever into the deepest possible twist. Let your heels come closer or completely, to the floor. Bring your left shoulder forward, your right shoulder back, and lift the chest. Don't lean back—lengthen forward and upward from the base of the spine. Keep the knees facing forward. Take a few breaths.

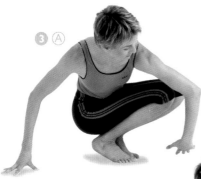

3 Ⓐ

and arm and wrap your arm behind your back to clasp the hands together. Ⓑ Look over the right shoulder, opening the chest to the side as much as possible.

4 After five breaths exhale, release the hands, and turn the trunk back to the front. Repeat on the other side.

3 Ⓑ

3 Stretch the left shoulder forward to bring the armpit in contact with the knee. Internally rotate the shoulder (so the elbow points forward), then bring the hand left under the shins. Ⓐ Take the hand close to the left hip. Bring your weight forward and lift the right hand off the floor. Internally rotate the right shoulder

INFORMATION

GAZE To the side.

BUILD-UP POSES Bound Sage Pose, Garland Pose, Revolved Chair Pose.

COUNTER POSES Deep Forward Fold, Garland Pose, East Stretch Posture.

LIGHTEN a) Place a folded blanket or a block under the heels to assist with

the balance. **b)** Bring the front hand to the floor near the toes to use it to lever your twist deeper. **c)** Grasp a belt in both hands to wrap the arms fully around the legs. **d)** Wrap the left arm around the left leg only, so the arm is between the knees. **e)** Do not go to the final (binding) stage.

EFFECT Opening.

Scales Pose

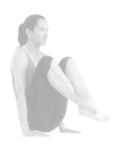

Tolasana In this continuation of Lotus Posture, the buttocks are lifted off the floor. This develops shoulder, arm, and abdominal strength. The true test of having mastered such a posture is when the lift off the floor becomes comfortable enough to be steadily sustainable.

1 Sit in Lotus Posture (page 152). Have the knees quite close together so the lotus is fairly "tight."

2 Place the hands on either side of the hips, fingers pointing forward. Press the hands down, then, with an exhalation, grip the *bandhas* strongly and lift the buttocks off the floor. Lift the knees up as close to the chest as possible.

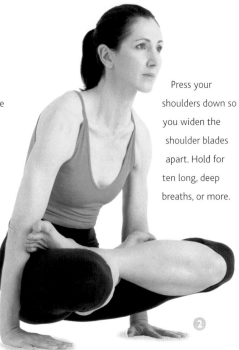

Press your shoulders down so you widen the shoulder blades apart. Hold for ten long, deep breaths, or more.

3 Exhale, lower the body, release the hands, then straighten the legs and repeat on the opposite side.

4 If your body is not ready for Lotus Posture, sit in a simple cross-legged pose instead (see Easy Seated Pose, page 106). Draw the knees up close to the trunk so you make your body as small a unit as possible. Activate your abdominal muscles. Press your hands to the floor just in front of your hips. Lean forward and then lift your buttocks and possibly your feet off the floor.

INFORMATION

GAZE Tip of nose.

BUILD-UP POSES Lotus Posture (and its preparations), Boat Pose, One Hand Over Arm Balance.

COUNTER POSES Mountain Pose 2 (in Hero Pose), Wrist Releases.

LIGHTEN a) From Easy Seated Pose, lift only the buttocks off the floor, leaving the feet on the floor.

EFFECT Strengthening.

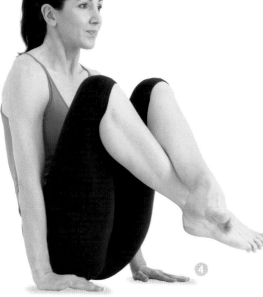

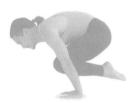

Pendant Pose

Lolasana In this dynamic posture, the body swings between the arms like a pendant on a necklace, developing strength in the shoulders and the abdominal muscles.

1 Kneel on the floor with the feet together so you are sitting on your heels. This is called Thunderbolt Pose.

2 With your hands on the floor tuck your toes under, and lean forward so that the shoulders are above the line of the fingertips and the knees are in front of the forearms. Press the hands down, lift the buttocks a little, and lift the knees off the floor.

3 Lean forward more, and using your abdominal muscles fully extend the

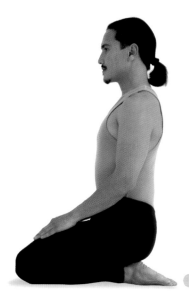

arms to draw the knees toward the chest. Make the body as compact as possible. Point the toes back as you balance on the hands. Spread your shoulder blades apart and push the floor away with the palms, spreading your weight evenly. Dangling like a pendant, swing back and forth a few times.

4 On an exhalation, lower the legs down, change the crossing of the ankles and repeat. Once this posture has been mastered, it is also possible to come into it from Easy Seated Pose (page 106) by lifting up and swinging the legs back.

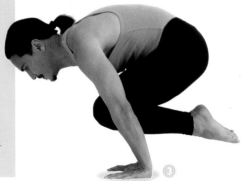

INFORMATION

GAZE Tip of nose.

BUILD-UP POSES Downward Facing Dog Pose, Boat Pose, Scales Pose, Arm Pressure Balance.

COUNTER POSES Mountain Pose 2 (in Head Pose), Wrist releases, East Stretch Posture.

LIGHTEN a) Raise the hands on foam or wooden blocks. **b)** Only lift the knees off the floor, leaving the feet lightly touching.

EFFECT Strengthening.

Half Lotus Heron Pose

Ardha Padma Krounchasana This pose gives an intense stretch to the back of the legs in an upright, seated position, with the added bonus of working the abdominal muscles strongly. This pose is very similar in form to Half Bound Lotus Forward Bend (page 146), just in a different relationship to gravity.

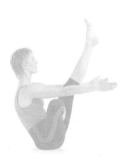

1 Sit on the floor with both legs extended in Seated Staff Posture (page 104). Bend the right knee out to the side and bring the right ankle on top of the left thigh. To avoid straining ligaments place the outer right ankle, rather than the side of the foot against the thigh. To avoid placing undue strain on the knee, the hips need to be ready for this position.

For hip opening preparations to help achieve this position, see Cow Posture (page 140) and Half Bound Lotus Forward Bend (page 146).

2 Bend the left knee in toward the chest and grasp the left heel with both hands. Ⓐ Keep pulling back on the heel as you straighten the leg up in the air. Lift the upper body

and the extended leg more to vertical. Bring the leg closer to your face. Ⓑ Press down into the sitting bone and draw in the lumbar spine in toward the navel to avoid rounding the lower back. Keep your shoulders relaxed as you stretch open the back of the extended leg.

❷ Ⓑ 3 After several breaths here, next firm the abdominal muscles in anticipation of releasing the leg. Draw the leg closer in,

release your grip and stretch the arms out parallel to the floor. Keep the leg up high. Hold for five breaths. Then exhale and move the leg down to the floor.

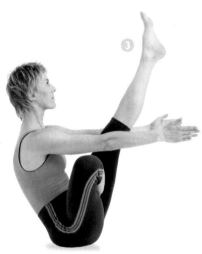

INFORMATION

GAZE Tip of nose.

BUILD-UP POSES Preparations from Cow Posture and Half Bound Lotus Forward Bend, Half Bound Lotus Forward Bend, Half Bound Lotus Stretch, Boat Pose.

COUNTER POSES Hero Pose, East Stretch Posture.

LIGHTEN a) Keep raised leg bent. **b)** Use a strap around foot of raised leg. **c)** Hold calf muscle or thigh of raised leg instead of heel. **d)** Place the sole or side of the foot of the bent leg on the floor.

EFFECT Strengthening.

Extended Leg Fish Pose

Uttana Padasana In this continuation of Fish Pose (page 262) the legs are kept straight and lifted off the floor. This pose increases abdominal strength and, by placing more pressure through the cervical vertebrae, protects them from loss of bone density. It follows well after Shoulderstand (page 286) and its variations.

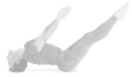

1 Lie on your back with the feet together. Straighten the arms alongside the body, and place the hands palms down under the buttocks. Press the elbows down and lift the chest off the floor. Still looking forward, go for your maximum lift. Push up through the sternum to lift the heart center. Tilt the head back, stretch the chin away, and rest the crown of the head on the floor in Fish Pose. Draw in the lumbar vertebrae toward the front of the body. With this increased concave shape in the lower back, bring the crown of the head closer to the sacrum,

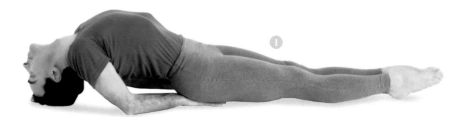

letting the head take the weight of the torso. Do not support the weight of the body with the arms.

2 Without moving the head or chest, lift the legs and extend them away. Now bring the palms together above the abdomen so that the arms are pointing upward at 45°, parallel to the legs. Keep the legs

and arms straight and stretch out the toes. The weight of the body will be resting only on the crown of the head and the buttocks.

3 Exhale, lower the legs and the arms, then release the head and rest on the floor.

INFORMATION

GAZE Tip of nose.

BUILD-UP POSES Fish Pose, Boat Pose, Hare Pose.

COUNTER POSES Supported Bridge Pose, Double Leg Forward Stretch, Neck Releases.

LIGHTEN a) Bend the knees. **b)** Bend the knees to help lift the legs in the air. **c)** Rest the tips of the toes lightly on the floor.

EFFECT Strengthening.

Arm Balances

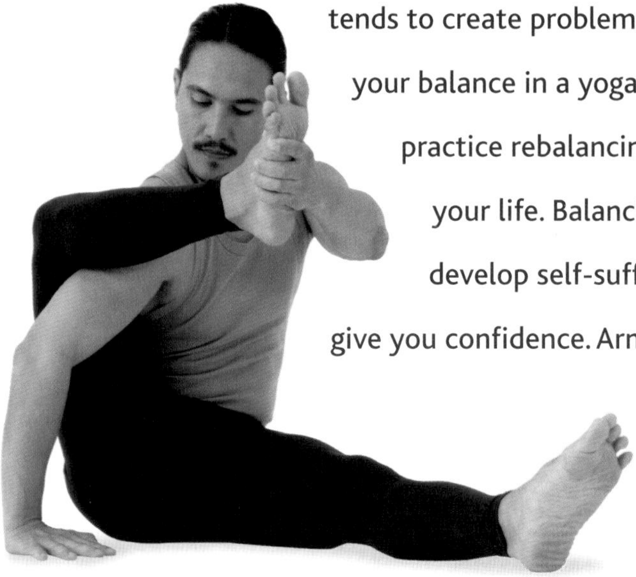

Being out of balance is a huge source of stress and

tends to create problems. Finding

your balance in a yoga pose lets you

practice rebalancing the rest of

your life. Balancing postures

develop self-sufficiency and

give you confidence. Arm balances,

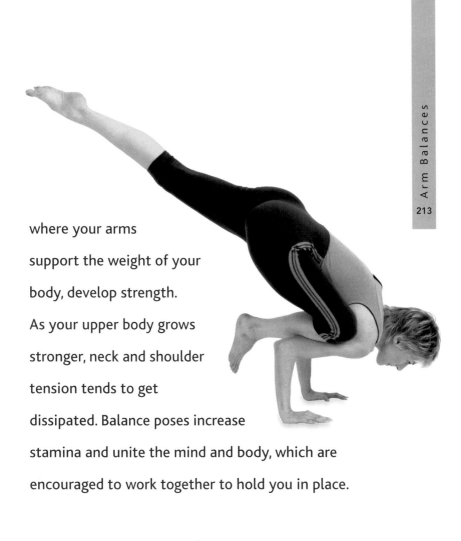

where your arms
support the weight of your
body, develop strength.
As your upper body grows
stronger, neck and shoulder
tension tends to get
dissipated. Balance poses increase
stamina and unite the mind and body, which are
encouraged to work together to hold you in place.

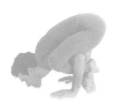

Arm Pressure Balance

Bhujapidasana This posture strengthens the wrists, arms, and shoulders. It also works the adductor muscles, which are used to press the legs against the arms.

1 Stand with the feet parallel, about 1 foot (30 centimeters) apart. Bend forward, lift the left heel, and thread the left arm between the legs to wedge the shoulder behind the left knee. Position the hand flat on the floor behind, just outside the left heel with the fingers pointing forward. The right hand lies forward.

2 Don't squat down too much—keep the buttocks high so you can then repeat the sequence with the right arm. Then rest the backs of the thighs as high as possible on the upper arms, as if sitting on the elbows.

3 Gradually lean back and transfer the weight of the body from the feet to the hands. Straighten the arms and balance on the hands. Lift the feet off the floor and

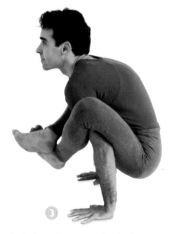

interlock the ankles. Press the thighs against the arms to prevent them from slipping down. Stay in this position for five to ten breaths. Alternate the crossing of the ankles each time you practice.

4 From here, advanced practitioners can exhale, bend the elbows, tilt the body forward, swing the feet back between the hands,

INFORMATION

GAZE Tip of nose.

BUILD-UP POSES Downward Facing Dog Pose, One Hand Over Arm Balance.

COUNTER POSES Mountain Pose 2 (in Hero Pose), Wrist Releases.

LIGHTEN a) Do not go to the final stage. **b)** Practice transferring weight from feet to hands. **c)** Use blocks under the hands. **d)** In the final stage, bring the crown of the head, rather than the chin, to the floor.

EFFECT Strengthening.

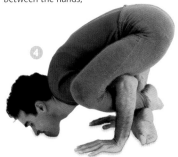

and lower the crown of the head, or, if possible, the chin toward the floor, looking forward. Work the abdominal muscles and do not allow the feet to touch the floor. Stay in this position for five to ten breaths. Inhale, swing back up, cross the ankles the other way, and repeat the posture.

Crane Posture

Bakasana In this posture, the whole weight of the body rests on the hands. This strengthens the wrists, arms, shoulders, and abdominal muscles. It requires concentration and, in helping us conquer the fear of falling forward, builds confidence in other areas of our life.

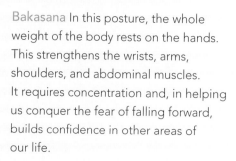

Stand in Mountain Pose (page 46). Squat down and place the hands flat on the floor, shoulder width apart, and about 10 inches (25 centimeters) in front of the feet, with the middle fingers pointing forward. With feet close together, come onto tiptoes, widen the knees and bend the elbows. Lift the heels higher and bring your weight forward to place the knees on the upper arms as

close to the armpits as possible. Continue to press the knees in against the upper arms.

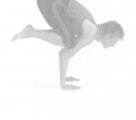

Slowly lean forward, transferring your body weight from the feet to the hands. Trust in the support of your arms as you let your face move forward. Once the weight is on the hands, lift the feet up and straighten the

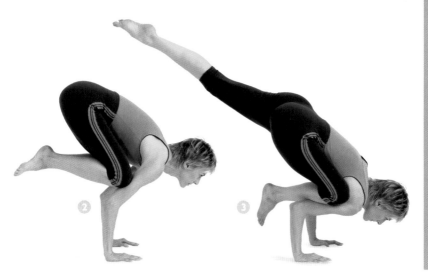

GAZE Tip of nose.

BUILD-UP POSES Downward Facing Dog Pose, Arm Pressure Balance.

COUNTER POSES Mountain Pose 2 (in Hero Pose), Camel Posture, Wrist Releases.

LIGHTEN a) Practice transferring weight back and forth from toes to palms. **b)** Do not straighten the arms, but learn first to balance with bent elbows. **c)** Use blocks under the hands.

EFFECT Strengthening.

arms as much as possible. Keep the feet together. To develop the wrist muscles and protect the wrists, "claw" the ground with the fingertips. This is Crane Posture. Stay here for five to ten breaths. Keep your concentration as you come out of the posture. Slowly bend the elbows, bring the feet back to the floor, and stand up.

3 From Crane Posture, advanced practitioners can bend the elbows more and straighten one leg back in the air to One Legged Crow Pose. Stay in this position for a few seconds, bend the raised leg back into Crane Posture position, and then repeat on the other side.

Inclined Plane Posture

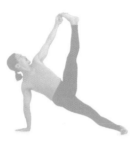

Vasisthasana This posture strengthens the wrists, arms, shoulders, and abdomen. The final stage also limbers the legs. You are likely to have all the strength you need to achieve the posture. Tap into the power of your mind to hold this pose steady.

1 Perform Downward Facing Dog Pose (page 162). Turn the heel of the right foot out and lay the outer edge of the foot down along the floor in a direct line back from the right hand. Take the left foot to the floor in front.

2 Let your body weight move forward toward your right hand as you transfer your weight onto it. To be able to lower the hips to have the body in one straight line, your right shoulder needs to be exactly above your right wrist, so, if necessary, return to Downward Facing Dog Pose and shorten or lengthen the distance between the hands and feet.

3 Place your left foot on top of the right foot and extend away through both heels. Turn the trunk to the left as you reach the left hand toward the sky. Don't sag the hips down—use your abdominal muscles to keep the whole body straight. Turn the head to look up at the left hand. Secure the balance and stay in this position for five to ten breaths.

4 Bend the top knee forward toward the chest and catch the big toe with the

index and the middle finger of the left hand. Straighten the arm and leg upward. If you can balance, turn the head and gaze at the big toe. Hold this position for five to ten breaths.

5 Exhale, lower the raised leg, release the toe and replace the right hand, then the feet back to stretch for a few breaths in Downward Facing Dog Pose. Repeat the posture on the other side.

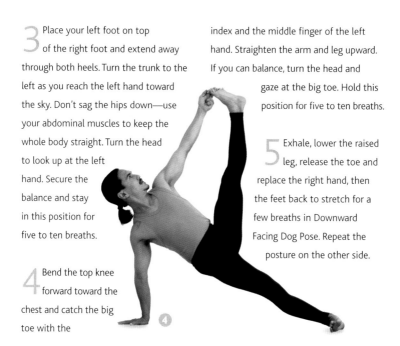

INFORMATION

GAZE Top hand.

BUILD-UP POSES Upright Big Toe Sequence, Reclining Hand to Toe Sequence, Downward Facing Dog Pose, Four Limbed Staff Pose.

COUNTER POSES Wrist Releases, Downward Facing Dog Pose, Child Pose.

LIGHTEN a) Bend the lower knee and rest that knee and shin on the floor, toes pointing back. **b)** Balance on the lower forearm rather than on the hand. **c)** Have the sole of the lower foot against a wall. **d)** Do not go to the final stage.

EFFECT Strengthening.

Inclined Plane Variations

Vasisthasana These advanced variations of Inclined Plane Posture (page 218) demand arm and shoulder strength. Mental focus is required, since they present a further challenge to your flexibility and balance.

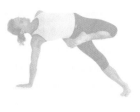

1 Begin in Inclined Plane Posture (page 218) and lay the top arm alongside the body. Keep the whole body straight.

2 Bend the top knee forward to the chest. Take hold of the foot with the top hand and extend the knee away to bring the heel close to the top buttock. Pressing the top of the foot forward, swivel the hand outward, bringing the elbow up and out, until the fingers are pointing away from the foot. Use your hand to press the foot forward to the side of the hip. Stay for five to ten breaths in Frog Inclined Plane Posture (shown from the opposite side).

INFORMATION

GAZE Tip of nose.

BUILD-UP POSES Inclined Plane Posture, Frog Pose, Half Lotus Pose preparations, Half Bound Lotus Pose.

COUNTER POSES Wrist Releases, Mountain Pose 2 (in Hero Pose), Double Leg Forward Stretch, Embryo Pose or (Extended) Child Pose.

LIGHTEN a) Bend the lower knee and rest that knee and shin on the floor, toes pointing back. **b)** Balance on the lower forearm rather than on the hand. **c)** Have the sole of the lower foot against a wall. **d)** Do not hold toes in Kasyapa Pose. **e)** Keep fingers pointing back in Frog Inclined Plane Posture.

EFFECT Strengthening, centering.

3 Exhale, release the leg, and with control come back to Downward Facing Dog Pose (page 162). Rest in Child Pose (page 100) if necessary, then repeat on the other side for the same length of time.

Plane Posture. Press the sole of the foot to the floor, then bend the top leg in. Bring the foot to the root of the supporting thigh in Half Lotus Pose (page 152). Swing the top arm behind the back and catch the toes of the lotus foot. Stay for five to ten breaths.

4 Kasyapa Pose is named after Kasyapa, a legendary sage, father of the gods and of the demons. For this pose, start with the basic Inclined

5 To come out of the pose, release the right foot, straighten the leg and come back to Downward Facing Dog Pose. Rest if necessary, then repeat on the other side.

▲

One Hand Over Arm Balance

Eka Hasta Bhujasana Having one leg extend away creates a heavy weight for the arms to lift. This posture develops strength in the wrists, arms, and shoulders. It also requires a great deal of abdominal strength.

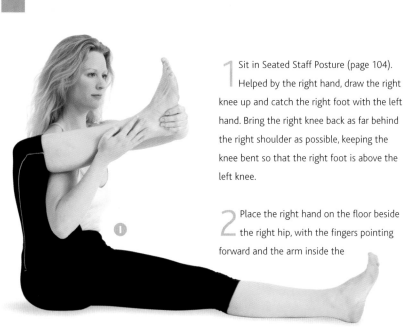

1 Sit in Seated Staff Posture (page 104). Helped by the right hand, draw the right knee up and catch the right foot with the left hand. Bring the right knee back as far behind the right shoulder as possible, keeping the knee bent so that the right foot is above the left knee.

2 Place the right hand on the floor beside the right hip, with the fingers pointing forward and the arm inside the

right knee. Place the left hand on the floor beside the left hip with the fingers pointing straight ahead. The key is to press the right calf strongly down against the arm, as if you were trying to squash the upper arm. With the elbows bent but not locked, press both hands strongly into the floor and lift the whole body up. Keep the left leg straight. Have it parallel to the floor, or, if possible, lift it higher. Press the right leg against the arm to prevent it from slipping down. Then stretch out the toes of both legs. Stay for five breaths or more with even breathing.

INFORMATION

GAZE Tip of nose.

BUILD-UP POSES Downward Facing Dog Pose, Arm Pressure Balance, Boat Pose.

COUNTER POSES Wrist Releases, Mountain Pose 2 (in Hero Pose), Forearm Releasing Forward Fold.

LIGHTEN a) Leave the left foot on the floor, only lifting the buttocks off the floor. **b)** Place the hands on blocks.

EFFECT Strengthening.

3 Exhale, lower the body down to the floor, release the right leg and straighten it, then repeat on the other side for the same length of time.

Eight Bend Balance

Astavakrasana This very strong twist strengthens the wrists, arms, and shoulders. It develops a sense of cooperation within the body as you find the delicate balance between letting yourself tip forward while your arms work strongly to keep you aloft.

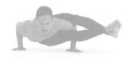

1 Sit on the floor with the knees bent up. Pick up your left leg, bend forward, and wrap it over your left arm. Your inner knee needs to sit high up on the arm, wedged behind the shoulder if possible.

2 Place the left hand flat on the floor just to the side and in front of the left buttock. Have the fingers pointing forward and bend the elbow so it pushes back strongly into the thigh to help keep the top knee in place. Place the right hand flat on the floor just in front and to the side of the right buttock. Interlock the ankles with the right ankle on top. At this stage both knees are bent.

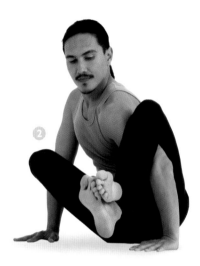

INFORMATION

GAZE Tip of nose.

BUILD-UP POSES Arm Pressure Balance, Scales Pose, One Hand Over Arm Balance.

COUNTER POSES Wrist Releases, Mountain Pose 2 (in Hero Pose), Double Leg Forward Stretch.

LIGHTEN a) Do not go to the final stage. **b)** Use blocks under the hands.

EFFECT Strengthening.

3 Gradually tip your body forward as you transfer its weight to the palms. Start to extend your legs away to the right as you lift the buttocks and bend the elbows deeply.

5 To come out of this posture, inhale, straighten the arms, bend the knees in, and sit back up. Release the legs, then repeat on the other side.

4 Your chin will come close to the floor and your trunk and the upper arms will be parallel to the floor. Keep a tension in your legs as if you were trying to straighten them. Stay in this position for five to ten breaths.

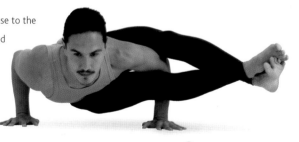

Firefly Balance

Tittibhasana Like all the arm balancing postures, Firefly Balance strengthens the wrists, arms, and shoulders. It also works into the hips and gives a very strong stretch to the hamstring muscles. This posture can be done as a continuation to Arm Pressure Balance (page 214).

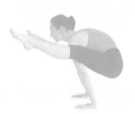

1 Stand with the feet parallel, about 1 foot (30 centimeters) apart. Bend forward and, one by one, take the arms between the legs to wedge the shoulders behind the knees. Place each hand flat on the floor behind and just outside the heels with the fingers pointing forward. To perform this posture properly the legs must be as high as possible on the arms.

2 Gradually lean back and transfer the weight of the body from the feet to the hands. Rest the back of the thighs on the upper arms, as if sitting on the elbows. Straighten the arms and balance on the hands.

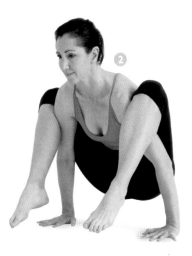

INFORMATION

GAZE Tip of nose.

BUILD-UP POSES Seated Angle Posture, Tortoise Posture, Crane Posture.

COUNTER POSES Wrist Releases, East Stretch Posture, Forearm Releasing Forward Fold.

LIGHTEN Use blocks under the hands.

EFFECT Strengthening.

3 Lift the feet off the floor and straighten the legs. At first it is difficult to straighten the legs in this position, so work on forward bends to release the hamstrings and this will become easier with practice. Press the legs against the arms. Point the toes and look straight ahead. Stay for five to ten breaths. Advanced practitioners can work at bringing the hips down and the feet up, so the legs become more vertical.

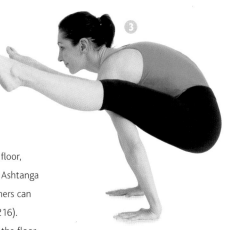

4 Exhale, bend the elbows, sit down on the floor, and relax. From Firefly Balance, advanced Ashtanga Vinyasa yoga (page 385). Some yoga practitioners can swing the legs back into Crane Posture (page 216). Otherwise, exhale, bend the elbows and sit on the floor.

One Legged Sage Balance 1

Eka Pada Galavasana This challenging hand-balancing posture strengthens the wrists and the arms, exercises the abdominal muscles and develops mental focus and staying power.

1 From standing, bring your left ankle high up on the right thigh, as close to the top of the thigh as possible. Squat down a little and fold forward to work into the right buttock muscles.

2 With the supporting leg bent, lean forward and bring your palms to the floor, shoulder width apart. Raise the right heel, lean forward more and bring the left foot around the right upper arm, just above the elbow. Flex the ankle to wrap the foot around the arm. Bring the left shin to the table-like left upper arm.

3 While learning this pose it might help to bring the crown of your head to the floor. Take more weight into the palms and lift the right foot off the floor, so your knee is in the

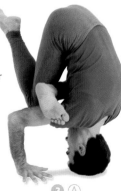

3 Ⓐ

3 **B**

air between the elbows. **A** Extend the right leg back in the air, then lift the head off the floor. Lift the back leg and the head as far up as possible.

B Work your back muscles to move the stretch evenly through the entire length of the spine. This is the final posture. Stay for five to ten breaths, then repeat on the other side.

4 Advanced practitioners can start in Tripod Pose (page 302). Bend the right knee and place the right foot at the root of the left thigh so it is in a Half Lotus Position (page 152). Bend the left knee down.

INFORMATION

GAZE Tip of nose.

BUILD-UP POSES Half Lotus Pose preparations, Tripod Pose, Crane Posture.

COUNTER POSES Child Pose, Wrist Releases, Forearm Releasing Forward Fold, Double Leg Forward Stretch.

LIGHTEN Do not lift the head off the floor.

EFFECT Strengthening.

5 Lower the legs so that the right shin rests on the back of the upper right arm and the right foot on the back of the upper left arm. Gradually lift the head off the floor and stretch the left leg back. Exhale, bend the left leg in, place the head back on the floor and lift back up into Tripod Pose, then repeat on the other side.

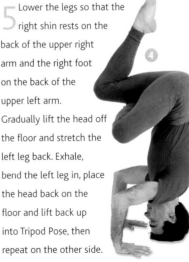

Sideways Crow Posture

Parsva Bakasana This balancing posture requires strength in the wrists, arms, shoulders, and abdominal muscles. As the abdominal muscles work strongly in a very active twist, it has a powerful toning effect on the abdominal organs.

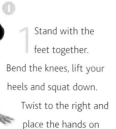

1 Stand with the feet together. Bend the knees, lift your heels and squat down. Twist to the right and place the hands on the floor to the side of your right foot in the same line as your shoulders. Have your palms flat on the floor at least 1 foot (30 centimeters) in front of the side of the right foot and a little wider than shoulder width apart. Have your torso as perpendicular to your thighs as possible.

2 Bend your left elbow to make a small shelf for your knees. Press your knees as high up as possible against the upper left arm and go as deeply as possible into your twist. Transfer your weight from the feet to the hands. Provided your hands are far enough forward, you will be able to lift your feet as your body moves forward.

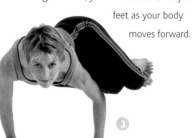

3 Pull the heels to the buttocks. Press the legs more against the upper arm. Resist with the upper arm to balance. Work the wrists by gripping the ground with the fingers so the fingertips go white.

4 This pose may also be entered from Tripod Pose (page 302). From your tripod, keep the knees and ankles together, bend the knees and bring the legs outside the left elbow. Swing the legs over as much as possible, so the side of the left thigh rests on the back, rather than the top, of the upper left arm. Gradually lift the head off the floor, at the same time pulling the feet up. Straighten the arms. Keep the weight equally distributed between the two hands.

5 After five to ten breaths, bend the arms, place the head back on the floor and come back up into Tripod Pose, then repeat on the other side.

INFORMATION

GAZE Tip of nose.

BUILD-UP POSES Crane Posture, Eight Bend Balance, Revolved Chair Pose, Tripod Pose.

COUNTER POSES Wrist Releases, Forearm Releasing Forward Fold, Double Leg Forward Stretch, East Stretch Posture.

LIGHTEN a) Practice transferring weight from the feet to the palms. **b)** When twisting right, place the right palm closer so instead of having that arm straight, you can rest the right hip on the bent right elbow, creating an easier table of support with both elbows. **c)** Entering from Tripod Pose, do not lift the head off the floor.

EFFECT Strengthening.

▲

One Legged Sage Balance 2

Eka Pada Koundinyasana This advanced balancing posture combines an arm balance with a twist. It strengthens the wrist and the arms, exercises the abdominal muscles, and massages the abdominal viscera.

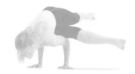

1 From Downward Facing Dog Pose (page 162), step the right leg forward and across to bring the right foot to the outside of the left hand.

2 Bend the left elbow slightly and place the outside of the right thigh as high as possible against the back of the upper left arm. You are in a sort of twisting lunge.

3 Gradually lean forward, bending the elbows and bringing the weight onto the hands. The right thigh will now be pressing against the upper left arm. Balance on the hands. At first it may be easier to rest the head on the floor.

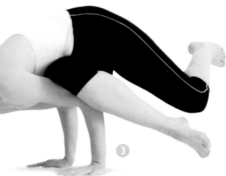

4 Stretch the right leg to the left and the left leg back. Lift the head and look forward. Keep the weight equally distributed between the two hands. Press the fingertips into the floor to protect the wrists. This is the final posture. Stay for five to ten breaths.

5 The traditional way of getting into the posture is to start in Tripod Pose (page 302). Then bend the knees and lower the right leg outside the left elbow. Swing the leg over as much as possible, so the side of the right thigh rests on the back, rather than the top, of the upper left arm. Stretch the right leg out to the left and the left leg straight back.

6 Gradually lift the head off the floor and look forward. Keep the legs straight. Stay in the final posture for five to ten breaths, then exhale, bend the arms and knees, place the head back on the floor, and come back up into Tripod Pose before repeating on the other side.

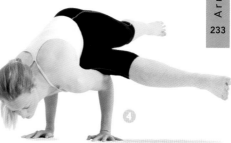

INFORMATION

GAZE Tip of nose.

BUILD-UP POSES Tripod Pose, Crane Posture, Sideways Crow Posture.

COUNTER POSES Downward Facing Dog Pose, Upward Facing Dog Pose, Double Leg Forward Stretch, Wrist Releases.

LIGHTEN a) Bend the right elbow as well as the left and use it to support the right hip. **b)** Keep the bottom leg bent. **c)** When entering from Headstand, do not lift the head off the floor.

EFFECT Strengthening.

Peacock Posture

Mayurasana This is a classic balancing posture, and great benefits are attributed to it in the classic yoga texts. The digestion and abdominal organs receive an increased blood supply due to the pressure of the elbows. It also strengthens the abdominal muscles and wrists.

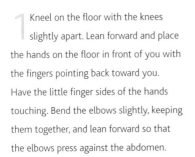

1 Kneel on the floor with the knees slightly apart. Lean forward and place the hands on the floor in front of you with the fingers pointing back toward you. Have the little finger sides of the hands touching. Bend the elbows slightly, keeping them together, and lean forward so that the elbows press against the abdomen.

2 Stretch the legs straight back so the weight of the body is resting on the wrists and the tops of the feet. Slowly move forward to transfer the weight of the body onto the hands and lift the feet off the floor. Lift the head and the legs to extend them away. Stay in this posture for five to ten breaths. The legs may be taken high in

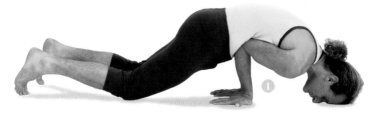

INFORMATION

GAZE Tip of nose.

BUILD-UP POSES Four Limbed Staff Pose, Locust Pose.

COUNTER POSES Wrist Releases, Mountain Pose 2 (in Hero Pose), Forearm Releasing Forward Fold,

Downward Facing Dog Pose.

LIGHTEN a) Have the hands slightly apart. **b)** Do not lift the feet off the floor.

EFFECT Strengthening.

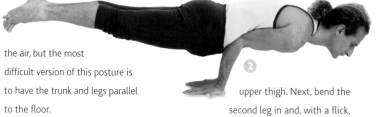

the air, but the most difficult version of this posture is to have the trunk and legs parallel to the floor.

3 Exhale, lower the feet and come back to kneeling.

4 A variation of this posture is done with the legs interlocked in Lotus Position (page 152). You need to have a well-established Lotus practice to master this. Once you are up and balancing on your hands bend one leg in and place the ankle on the

upper thigh. Next, bend the second leg in and, with a flick, place ankle on thigh to form the full lotus. This is called Lotus Peacock Posture. Each time you practice it, alternate the crossing of the legs.

Backbends

Backbends warm the system, increase energy, and invigorate us. They bring flexibility to our central axis of support and strengthen weak back muscles. Backbends counterpose the forward bending that dominates the day for many of us—sitting, driving, housework, and working at a desk. Backbends increase determination and willpower.

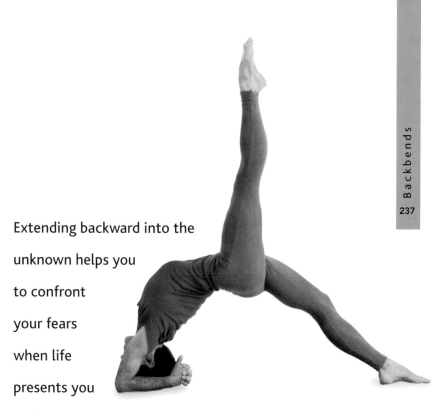

Extending backward into the unknown helps you to confront your fears when life presents you with an unknown quantity. Backbends open the chest, so they are uplifting. Opening the chest promotes better breathing and the heart center expands to bring a joyful vitality into your life.

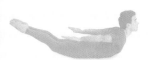

Locust Pose

Salabhasana This pose is particularly strengthening for the lower back muscles. It opens the chest, encourages good breathing, and dissipates mental fatigue.

1 Lie on your belly on the floor, legs extended and inner ankles touching. Allow the forehead to rest on the floor, so the back of the neck is long. Extend the arms beside the body, hands beside the hips and backs of the hands on the floor.

2 Soften the whole front of the body, surrendering to the support the floor is offering. Gently squeeze the buttocks together, rolling the thighs inward as you press the pubic bone toward the floor.

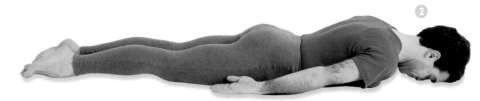

INFORMATION

GAZE Third eye or upward to infinity.

BUILD-UP POSES Cobra Pose, Sphinx Pose, Crocodile Pose.

COUNTER POSES Double Leg Forward Stretch. Lie on back and hug knees to chest.

LIGHTEN a) Alternate lifting just the legs, then just the upper body before lifting them both together. **b)** Keep the hands palms down on the floor beside the thighs. Press through the palms as you lift the chest.

EFFECT Invigorating, strengthening.

3 Extend through the arms, stretching the fingertips toward the feet, drawing the shoulders down the back, and opening across the front of the chest.

4 Inhale as you lift the chest and legs off the floor, keeping the shoulders unhunched and plenty of length in the back of the neck.

5 Lift the hands and wrists as you extend the fingertips back toward the feet. Breathe here for a few breaths. Even as you look up, tuck the chin in toward the chest a little to keep the neck and shoulders soft and relaxed.

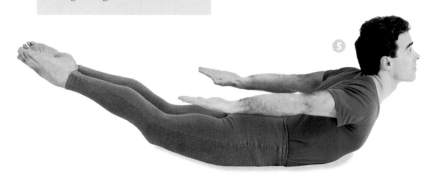

Sphinx Pose

Bhujangasana II This prone backbend
lifts the curve of the spine from the lower
back upward to the thoracic area. The
upper body bends backward less easily
than the lower back. This pose releases the
shoulders and opens the heart center.
It is a lovely stretch for the front of the body.

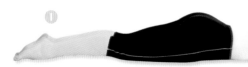

1 Lie face down on the floor. Stretch
both arms along the floor in front of
you, palms down. Then spread the fingers
wide. Have your legs straight with inner
thighs, knees, and ankles touching. Allow
the front of your body to begin to soften
and melt into the floor. Extend from the
shoulders through to the elbows. Then
lengthen from the elbows to the wrists
and out through each and every fingertip.

2 Inhale as you lift your head and
chest and slide the arms back toward
the body until the elbows are directly
beneath the shoulders. Roll the shoulders
back and pull them down, so they move
away from the ear lobes. As you extend
the spine upward, draw your shoulder
blades in closer toward the lungs.
Lengthen the lower back by pressing
the tailbone down toward the floor.

3 Press the forearms and palms of the hands evenly into the floor. Lengthen from the elbows to armpits as you "pull" your chest forward toward your fingertips so the side ribs move through the upper arms. Spread the backbend evenly through the back, so the middle and upper back curve more.

4 With eyes soft, gaze directly ahead into the vastness of infinity as you breathe into the heart space at the front of the chest. Release on an exhalation, turning your head to one side to rest your cheek on the floor. Allow yourself to be fully present with any sensations you may be experiencing. Repeat twice more.

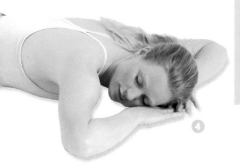

INFORMATION

GAZE Straight ahead.

BUILD-UP POSES Crocodile Pose, Locust Pose.

COUNTER POSES Embryo Pose, Child Pose.

LIGHTEN a) Cup the chin in the hands, with elbows on floor.
b) Keep more of your abdomen in contact with the floor.
c) Place the elbows forward of the shoulders.

EFFECT Energizing.

Cobra Pose

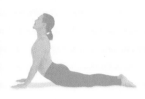

Bhujangasana I This backbend demands more arm strength than Sphinx pose. It opens the chest, stimulates the digestive organs, and increases mobility in the vertebral column.

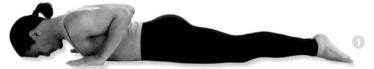

1 Lie face down on the floor. Place the palms on the floor under the shoulders, fingers facing forward. Over several releasing exhalations, make your body as long and alive as possible, extending from the back of the waist down through the lower back, hips, buttocks, thighs, calves, and soles of the feet.

2 Tuck your tailbone under so the pubic bone presses to the floor. Lift your straight knees off the floor while keeping the tops of the feet pressing down to the

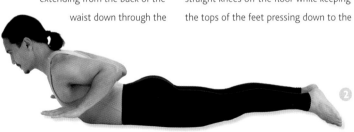

floor. Inhale and lift the chest upward without using any pressure at all on the palms. Hold for a few breaths. This position works on *strengthening* the back. It will give you an idea of which muscles you need to work, and how strong they are without any help from the arms.

3 Now work on *mobilizing* the back. Press the palms to the floor and continue to curl the spine up off the floor. Keep the inner legs and feet together as you press the pubic bone into the floor and move the back arching action a little higher up into the middle back. Pull back with the heels of the hands, so it feels like you are pulling your chest forward, through the arms.

4 Keep the shoulders soft and move down the back as you straighten the arms. Tuck the chin in toward the throat so the back of

INFORMATION

GAZE Third eye or upward to infinity.

BUILD-UP POSES Garland Pose, Warrior Pose 1.

COUNTER POSE Deep Forward Fold, Resting Deep Forward Fold.

LIGHTEN a) Practice moving smoothly in and out of the pose before holding it for longer periods.

EFFECT Energizing, strengthening.

the neck remains long. Stay here for a few more breaths, expanding the chest on the inhalation and lengthening the spine on the exhalation.

5 When you combine this pose with a hissing sound on each inhalation and an awareness of the line of energy from the perineum to the sacrum, it becomes a *mudra*, Serpent Seal.

Upward Facing Dog Pose

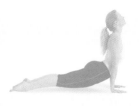

Urdhva Mukha Svanasana This posture strengthens the wrists and shoulders, opens the chest, and works the whole spine. It is one of the postures of the Sun Salutation sequence (page 42).

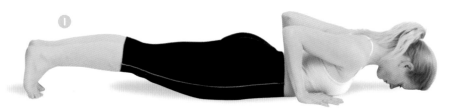

1 Lie on your stomach on the floor. Place the hands palms down by the side of the body so that the fingers point forward and are in line with the shoulders. Keep the elbows close to the body. Have the feet hip width apart. Tuck the toes under.

2 Inhale, press the palms into the floor, and lift the body off the floor slightly. With the help of the hands and feet, drag the hips forward as you roll forward over the toes so the tops of the feet are resting on the floor. Straighten the arms and lift the chest forward. Keep the legs straight and active. Activate your front thigh muscles to lift the knees off the floor, but keep the

GAZE Third eye or tip of nose.

BUILD-UP POSES Locust Pose, Cobra Pose.

COUNTER POSES Downward Facing Dog Pose, Double Leg Forward Stretch.

LIGHTEN a) Bend the knees slightly and rest them on the floor. **b)** Lift the hips higher if you have lower back pain.

EFFECT Opening, rejuvenating.

with the arms is that of dragging the hands back toward your hips (but without actually moving the palms). This helps your side ribs move forward through the upper arms so the chest will open farther. Tilt the head back gently and look up.

4 On an exhalation, bend the knees and come down.

5 Another way to exit the posture is to roll back over the toes with an exhalation, lifting the hips back, into Downward Facing Dog Pose (page 162), as in the Sun Salutation B sequence (page 42).

buttocks fairly relaxed. The weight of the body rests only on the top of the feet and on the palms of the hands.

3 Roll the shoulders down and back, keeping the chest lifting forward and up. The muscular action

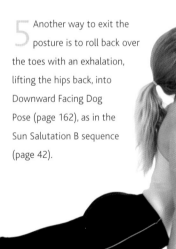

Crocodile Pose

Nakrasana While most backbends are outward-looking, this one allows the thoughts to turn inward as you rest. When you are building up to more and more difficult backbends, resting in Crocodile Pose is a good way to take a break without creating a counter pose to your sequence by rounding the back.

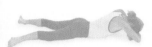

1 Lie face down on the floor. Inhale as you lift your head and chest and slide the arms back toward the body to bring the elbows in front of the shoulders.

2 Open the legs wide apart and roll the heels in, so that the inner thighs, knees, and ankles are in contact with the floor. Lengthen the tailbone toward the heels, gently squeeze the buttocks together and press the pubic bone into the floor.

3 Let the belly be soft as you lengthen the front of the body from the navel to the throat. Create space in the lumbar spine.

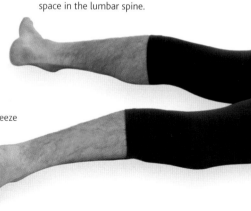

4 Lift the chest a little more as you bend the forearms in toward each other, cupping each elbow in a palm.

5 Tuck your chin into the throat so the back of the neck stays long. Rest your forehead on your forearms. You may need to reposition your elbows slightly forward or back so that your forehead comfortably rests down. Stretch the whole front of the body, from the inner edge of the feet, up through the inner thighs, pelvis, belly, and chest. Stay and quietly breathe. Release on an exhalation, turning the head and resting one cheek on the floor.

INFORMATION

GAZE Eyes closed.

BUILD-UP POSE Cobra Pose and Sphinx Pose, Locust Pose.

COUNTER POSE Embryo Pose, Child Pose, Extended Child Pose.

LIGHTEN a) Bring legs closer together. **b)** Move the elbows farther forward. **c)** Press less with the elbows.

EFFECT Restful, intuitive.

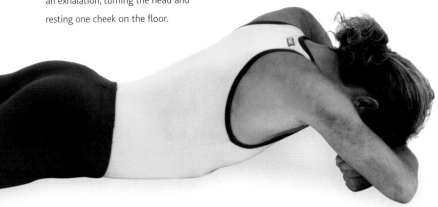

5

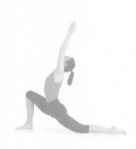

Crescent Moon Pose

Anjaneyasana This posture stretches the muscles at the front of the thighs, including the deep iliopsoas muscle, which is tight in many people. This intense backbend tones the kidneys and liver.

1 From a kneeling position, step the right foot forward with the knee bent so that the right thigh is parallel to the floor.

2 Extend through the front of the left leg. Stretch from the hip down to the knee. Extend from the knee to the ankle, then along the front of the foot through to the tips of the toes. With hands on the front knee, take the lunge deeper as you bend more into the right knee, so you feel the stretch in the front left thigh.

3 Raise both arms above the head, stretching all the way through to the fingers as you lift the chest. Have the intensity of the backbend comfortable enough so that you can lengthen the tailbone down toward

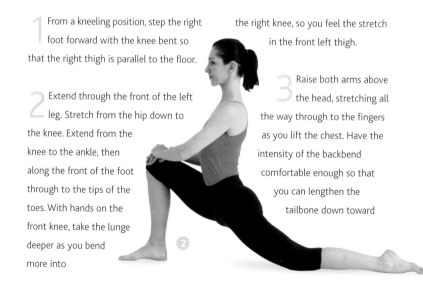

the floor to increase the stretch on the front of the left thigh. Let the hips drop down another notch. Now increase your backward bend to your personal maximum.

4 The lower back is the part that naturally curves most deeply. Consciously bring

the curve of the spine higher up into the middle back as you gracefully extend the arms back overhead and press your chest forward and up. Have your palms facing each other, or, if it doesn't create tightness in the neck or shoulders, press your palms together.

5 Turn your face to the sky and direct your gaze upward. Stay here for a few breaths, enjoying the crescent shape that you are in. On an exhalation, release the hands back to the floor to come onto all fours. Repeat on the other side.

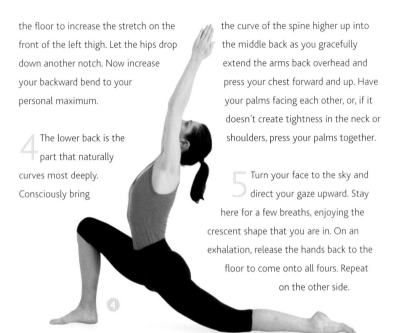

INFORMATION

GAZE Hands.

BUILD-UP POSES Cat Pose, Locust Pose, Cobra Pose, Bow Pose, Half Frog Pose, Reclining Half Hero Pose.

COUNTER POSES Child Pose, Cat Pose, Head Beyond the Knee Pose.

LIGHTEN a) Keep the fingertips beside front foot or on the front knee and follow the same instructions for backbending. **b)** Lunge less deeply into the front knee. **c)** Keep the front knee directly above the ankle. **d)** Pad under the back knee if necessary.

EFFECT Engaging.

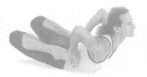

Frog Pose

Bhekasana This posture helps make the legs, particularly the knees, more flexible, stretches the quadriceps and iliopsoas muscles, while strengthening the arms.

1 Lie face down on the floor. Lift up the shoulders and bring the left arm across so that the elbow is underneath your left shoulder, and your hand underneath the right elbow. Bend your right knee and catch the top of the right foot with the right hand. Have your toes pointed straight forward, rather than out to the side.

2 On an exhalation, press the foot forward and down, then rotate the fingers of the right hand outward while bringing the elbow up and out until the fingers are pointing forward. With the elbow pointing up to the sky, press the foot down with the palm of the hand, so that the

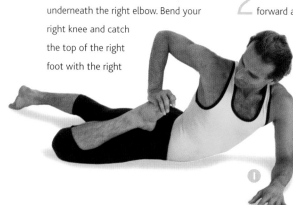

4 Now proceed to the full pose. Bend both knees and bring both heels close to the hips. Hold both feet with the hands. Rotate the hands as before and press the feet down, while lifting the chest off the floor and rolling the shoulders back.

Minimize how far apart the knees spread. Keep the elbows pulled in. Lift out of your waist to increase the backbend and create space in the abdomen and chest. Spread the backbend to include the stiffer parts of the spine. Relax the shoulders and neck. Stay for five to ten slow breaths.

2 inner heel scrapes the side of the buttock and hip, rather than the center of the buttock cheek. If possible, bring the heel to the floor. This is Half Frog Pose. Stay for five to ten breaths.

3 To increase the stretch on the front thigh stretch, press your right groin down to the floor and if possible lift the bent knee. Anchor down through the left elbow to deepen the curve in the upper back. Exhale, release the right foot and straighten the right leg, then repeat on the other side.

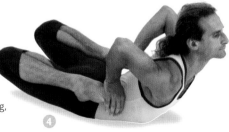

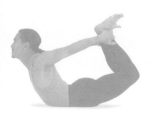

Bow Pose

Dhanurasana In this posture, the arms
are like the string of a bow, pulled tight
by the strength of the body and legs.
Bow Pose makes the spine flexible and
tones the abdominal organs. It can also
help relieve backache.

1 Lie face down on the floor. Bend both
knees to bring the heels close to the
buttocks. Reach back with the hands to
grasp the outer ankles. Do not widen the
knees; keep them no wider than the hips.
Start with your forehead on the floor.
Inhale and press the feet back and upward
so they lift away from your buttocks. Lift
your thighs as high as possible off the floor.

2 Now lift the head and chest up
as high as you can. Keep
the arms straight and pull
the shoulders back with the

strength of the legs. To increase the
roundedness of your bow, pull back on
the feet with the hands at the same time.
This action is as if you wanted to bend the
elbows, but because the feet are resisting
you won't be able to. Tilt the
head back and look up.
The weight of the

INFORMATION

GAZE Tip of nose.

BUILD-UP POSES Locust Pose, Reclining Hero Pose, Crescent Moon Pose.

COUNTER POSES Child Pose, Embryo Pose.

LIGHTEN a) Widen the knees apart.

b) Do not do Sideways Bow Pose.
c) If reaching the feet with the hands is difficult, use a belt around the feet.
d) Only do one side at a time (this is called Half Bow Pose).

EFFECT Energizing.

body should rest on the abdomen only. Stay for five to ten slow breaths. You may find that a rocking action occurs naturally in time with your breath.

floor. Stay for five breaths; then, on a strong inhalation, roll back to Bow Pose and repeat the posture on the other side.

3 For Sideways Bow Pose exhale and roll over to the right till the right shoulder and foot are on the floor and you are resting on the right side of the body. Stretch the abdomen and left hip forward while the feet press back. Turn the head to the left side and look up. Keep the right ear off the

4 Exhale, lower the legs and chest, and release the feet.

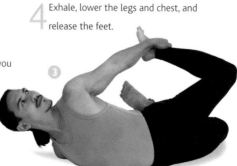

Gheranda Pose

Sukha Gherandasana This posture is
a combination of Bow Pose (page 252) on
one side and Frog Pose (page 250) on the
other side. It brings flexibility to the spine
and stretches the thigh muscles. The
pressure of breathing into the abdomen
pressing against the floor gives a good
massage to the abdominal organs.

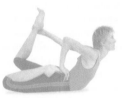

1 Lie face down on the floor. Bend the
right knee and take the foot beside the
right hip with the foot in line with the
shin, toes pointing straight forward. Catch
the foot with the right hand and, with an
exhalation, press the foot forward and
down, at the same time rotating the hand
outward, bringing the elbow out and up,
until the fingers are pointing forward.
Aim the foot toward the floor so it scrapes
the side of the hip on the way down.

2 Bend the left knee and reach back the
left hand to hold the left ankle. Inhale
and lift the left foot and the chest as high
as you can, at the same time pressing the
right foot down toward the floor with the
palm of the right hand. Do not roll over to
the right, but keep the hips

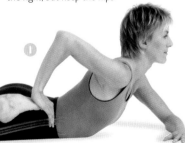

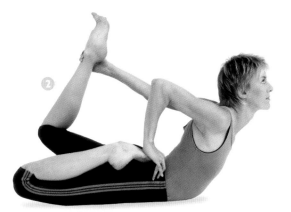

level. Keep the left arm straight and pull
the shoulders back with the strength of the
left leg. Tilt the head back and look up.
The weight of the body should rest on
the abdomen only. Raise the breastbone

up more to lift one more rib up off the
floor. Stay for ten slow, deep breaths.

3 Exhale, release the legs and repeat
on the other side.

INFORMATION

GAZE Tip of nose.

BUILD-UP POSES Bow Pose, Frog
Pose, Reclining Hero Pose, Cobra
Pose.

COUNTER POSES Child Pose,
Embryo Pose, Extended Child Pose.

LIGHTEN a) Practice only the left or
right side at once. **b)** With one side in
Bow or Frog, stretch the hand of the
opposite side forward while extending
the leg back and away, possibly lifting
both off the ground. **c)** Practice Bow
Pose and Frog Pose.

EFFECT Energizing.

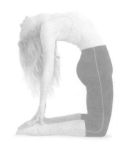

Camel Posture

Ustrasana This is an important posture, as it prepares the body and the mind for more difficult backbending postures. It limbers the shoulders, opens the chest, and makes the lower back flexible.

1 Kneel with the feet and knees together, the thighs and the body vertical. Have the tops of the feet on the floor so the toes point back. Place the hands on the hips, thumbs turned toward the spine and lift the torso from the base of the spine and pelvis, opening the chest. Don't collapse into your lower back—tuck your tailbone under and let the front of the thighs lengthen. Lift your collarbone higher. Squeeze your shoulder blades together as you roll the shoulders back. Arch your back.

2 Draw the abdominal muscles in toward the vertebral column. This protects the lower back while allowing the upper back to open deeply. While maintaining this muscle tension, move the hands away from the hips and reach back with the arms. Slowly drop back, reaching for the

2 heels with the hands, eventually placing the palms on the soles of the feet, fingers pointing back. Roll the shoulders back and lift up the lower ribs, arching the back as much as possible. Press the hips forward, so that the thighs are vertical. Relax the buttocks. Tilt the head back without tensing the neck. Stretch the chin away. Stay for five to ten slow breaths.

3 Ground through the knees and inhale strongly to come up, lifting the pelvis with the strength of the buttock muscles. To finish, sit down on the feet.

INFORMATION

GAZE Tip of nose.

BUILD-UP POSES Bow Pose, Cobra Pose, Crescent Moon Pose.

COUNTER POSES Child Pose, Head Beyond the Knee Pose.

LIGHTEN a) Tuck your toes under. **b)** Have the knees and feet hip width apart. **c)** Have someone help you by supporting you between the shoulder blades as you go back. **d)** Take one hand back at a time. **e)** Keep the head up, face looking forward.

EFFECT Energizing.

East Stretch Posture

Purvottanasana This posture strongly stretches the front of the body. In India, yoga is traditionally practiced facing East, so the front of the body is its East side, hence the name. It strengthens the wrist and arms and limbers the shoulders. It is an obvious counter pose to the seated forward bends.

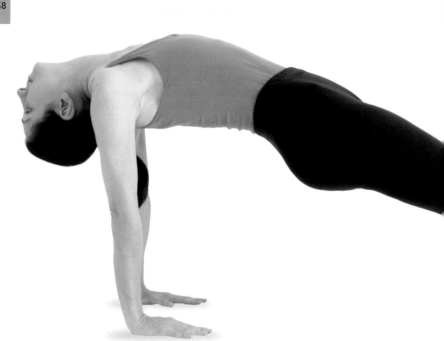

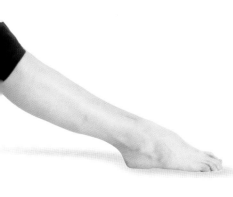

INFORMATION

GAZE Tip of nose.

BUILD-UP POSE Upward Facing Dog Pose.

COUNTER POSES Downward Facing Dog Pose, Double Leg Forward Stretch.

LIGHTEN a) Keep the knees bent. **b)** Place the feet closer and keep the knees at a right angle so you form a table-like shape.

EFFECT Energizing.

1 Sit in Seated Staff Posture (page 104). Place the hands shoulder width apart, 6 inches (15 centimeters) behind the back, with the fingers pointing toward the feet. Inhale, press the hands down, and lift the buttocks, taking the weight of the body on the hands and feet. Straighten the arms and lift the hips as high as possible. Straighten the legs and press the toes down toward the floor. Keep the heels and toes together and the thighs rotating inward.

2 The arms should be perpendicular to the floor while the torso arches upward. (Do not allow the hips to sag downward.) Still looking down the body, lift the hips until you can't see your toes. Then lift the chest until you can't see your hips. Gently tilt the head back, looking behind you and stretch the chin away. Broaden the chest. Press the floor away with the palms.

3 Stay in the posture for five to ten slow breaths, then exhale and come back down to Seated Staff Posture.

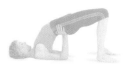

Bridge Pose

Setu Bandhasana This backbend strengthens and opens the chest, hips, lumbar spine, and fronts of the thighs. It works the nervous system to invigorate the whole body.

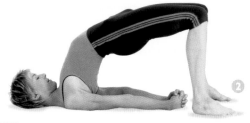

1 Lie on your back on the floor, arms beside you and knees bent. Place the feet hip width apart, heels in line with the sitting bones and toes pointing straight forward, rather than out to the sides. Press strongly into both feet as you inhale and lift the hips, raising the buttocks off the floor.

2 With the arms extended toward the feet, bring the palms of the hands together behind the back, interlocking the fingers. Press the little finger side of the hands against the floor as you extend the

knuckles toward the heels and lift the hips higher, rolling up onto the top of the shoulders. Tuck the chin in toward the chest, keeping the back of the neck long. Press up through the front of the thighs. Move your tailbone toward your knees. Take your knees closer together so they track forward over the toes. This is Bridge Pose.

3 If you have enough height, you'll be able to do the following variation.

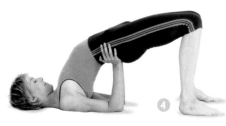

Keep the hips raised and unclasp the hands. Lean right, come onto the right toe tips, and bend the right forearm up to take right palm to the sacrum. Then repeat on the left side.

4 Lower both heels to the floor and reestablish the lift of your sternum and pubic bone. Bring the elbows toward each other, pressing the upper arms against the floor. Have the thumbs pressing along the spine as the fingers spread wide toward the hips. This is Supported Bridge Pose.

5 To take it one step further, try one legged Bridge Pose. Bring your feet together. Lean a little left, press the sole of the left foot strongly into the floor as you inhale, and lift the bent right leg off the floor. Extend the right foot toward the ceiling to vertical. Stay up for four to eight breaths, lifting the hips high and extending through the right foot. Release the right foot back to the floor on an exhalation. Repeat on the other side.

INFORMATION

GAZE Navel.

BUILD-UP POSES Locust Pose, Cobra Pose, Camel Posture, Bow Posture, Frog Pose.

COUNTER POSES Hug knees to chest and rock from side to side, Fish Pose, Revolved Abdomen Pose, Hare Pose, Head Beyond the Knee Pose, Neck Releases.

LIGHTEN a) Stay at the first stage. **b)** Rather than holding a long time, inhale up into the poise, then exhale down several times. **c)** For support at the second stage, use a block under the sacrum.

EFFECT Strengthening, opening.

Fish Pose

Matsyasana This pose honors Matsya, the incarnation of the Hindu god Vishnu as a fish. It is a backbend that strongly opens the chest and throat. It requires some flexibility in the thoracic spine. People with neck problems need to take care, as the neck is tightly flexed when the crown of the head is on the floor.

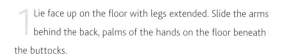

1 Lie face up on the floor with legs extended. Slide the arms behind the back, palms of the hands on the floor beneath the buttocks.

2 Press the forearms into the floor, and keep the elbows close together as you lift the upper arms and shoulders and arch up the chest. Gaze forward and allow the head to lift, continuing the upward arc of the chest into the throat. Move the chin away to stretch the throat.

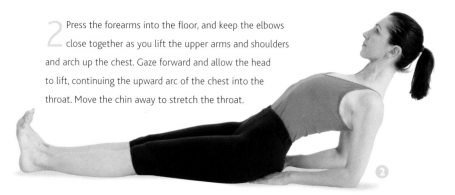

INFORMATION

GAZE Third eye.

BUILD-UP POSES Camel Posture, Cobra Pose, Supported Bridge Pose.

COUNTER POSES Hug knees to chest and rock side to side, Neck Releases, Plank Pose, Garland Pose.

LIGHTEN a) Don't drop the head back. **b)** Start from sitting: From Seated Staff Posture lean back on your hands or elbows as you lift your chest to recreate the back arching of Fish Pose.

EFFECT Uplifting.

Tilt the crown of the head back to rest lightly on the floor by widening your elbows apart. The key here is to really to lift up out of your lower back and press your breastbone up to the sky. When your chest is lifted enough, you will be able to choose how much pressure to place on the crown of your head against the floor.

3 Push the breastbone up to increase the arch from the pubic bone to the throat. Squeeze the shoulder blades together to take the shoulders down as you once again lift the chest. Press the inner legs together. Breathe deeply along the front of the body, enjoying the expanded openness of this pose.

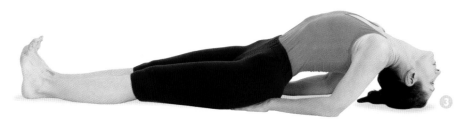

Bridge Posture

Setu Bandhasana In this posture the weight of the body rests entirely on the crown of the head and on the feet, with the legs and body forming a bridge. However, it puts extreme pressure on the cervical spine and should not be attempted by people who have problems or weakness in that area.

1 Lie on your back. Bend the knees outward and bring the heels about 2 feet (60 centimeters) away from the buttocks. The heels should be touching and the toes pointing outward at 45°. Lift the chest and arch the back as much as possible, and bring the crown of the head on the floor as in Fish Pose (page 262).

2 Take the palms to the floor on either side of the ears, to take some of the weight off the head when coming up into the posture. Now exhale and lift the hips as high as possible, balancing on the feet and the crown of the head. Slowly straighten the legs and roll the head back, trying to bring the forehead, or even the nose, to the floor. This puts considerable pressure on the cervical spine and can be challenging at first. Ⓐ

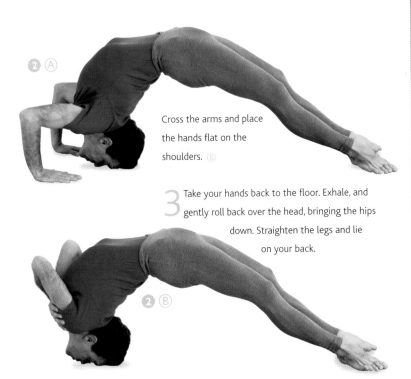

Cross the arms and place the hands flat on the shoulders. Ⓑ

3 Take your hands back to the floor. Exhale, and gently roll back over the head, bringing the hips down. Straighten the legs and lie on your back.

INFORMATION

GAZE Tip of nose.

BUILD-UP POSES Fish Pose, Camel Posture.

COUNTER POSES Neck Releases, Supported Bridge Pose, Double Leg Forward Stretch.

LIGHTEN a) Hold the side of the mat with straight arms. **b)** Lengthen the distance between the turned out feet and the buttocks. **c)** Do not straighten the legs fully.

EFFECT Energizing.

Upward Facing Bow Pose

Urdhva Dhanurasana This tremendous backbend engages every muscle in the body. It opens the front of the body strongly while giving the spine a maximum stretch. To lift into it requires good shoulder flexibility and, once up, strength in the arms to hold you in place.

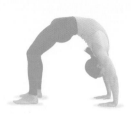

1 Lie on your back on the floor. Bend your knees and bring your heels up to your buttocks. Make sure the soles of the feet are spread firmly across the floor. The feet and, in particular, your heels are your foundation while you are in the pose. Bring the palms to the floor beside the shoulders, with the elbows pointing up and the fingers stretching toward your feet.

2 Lift your hips off the floor. Consolidate here for a while. Wait for an internal message telling you that you are ready to rise up. Then inhale, push strongly into the palms, and lift the head up, then tilt it backward to bring the crown of the head lightly to the floor. Stay here for a couple of breaths, adjusting to the feeling of being upside down and gathering your strength to raise your whole body off the floor.

upward arch with the front of the body, feeling a stretch all the way from the inner wrists along the forearms, along the sternum, through the abdomen and running down the front of the thighs to the feet. Get a sense of length through the back side of the body too.

3 On a new inhalation, push the floor away with your palms and the soles of the feet and lift up to an arch. Extend through the arms so they are as straight as possible. Allow the head to hang, gazing down toward the hands.

5 To come down, exhale, bend the arms and lower the crown of your head to the floor. On a new exhalation tuck the chin in, bend the arms and the knees, and lower the back to the floor. Rest for a few breaths before repeating twice more. Finish with a counter pose.

4 Stay up for five to ten breaths. Keep the elbows straight and work the knees straighter as you press open the front of the body. Make an

INFORMATION

GAZE Tip of nose.

BUILD-UP POSES Supported Bridge Pose, Bow Pose, Crescent Moon Pose, Reclining Hero Pose, Downward Facing Dog Pose.

COUNTER POSES Child Pose, Head Beyond the Knee Pose, Double Leg Forward Stretch.

LIGHTEN a) Do not go to final stage.

EFFECT Energizing.

Inverted Staff Posture

Dvi Pada Viparita Dandasana In this posture the weight of the body rests on the head, forearms, and feet. It increases flexibility in the entire spine, particularly the lumbar area, and is very exhilarating.

1 Lie on your back. Bend the knees and bring the feet close to the buttocks, hip width apart. Place the hands on either side of the head with the fingers pointing toward the feet. Take a few preparatory breaths. Lift the hips up and, when you are ready, inhale up into Upward Facing Bow Pose (page 266).

2 Take several breaths here, spreading the backbend evenly through the spine.

If you feel you need more warming up, come down to lie on the floor and repeat Upward Facing Bow Pose twice more.

3 Now lower the crown of the head to the floor. One by one, move the hands to behind the head, taking the elbows to the floor. Interlock the fingers so the hands cradle the back of the head as in

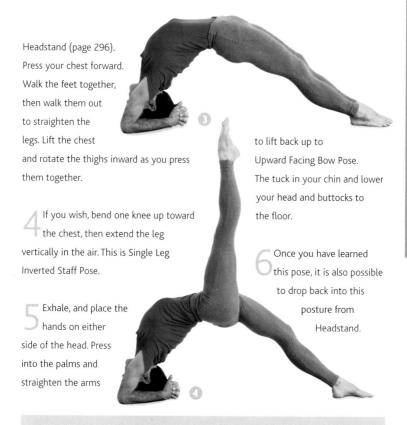

Headstand (page 296). Press your chest forward. Walk the feet together, then walk them out to straighten the legs. Lift the chest and rotate the thighs inward as you press them together.

4 If you wish, bend one knee up toward the chest, then extend the leg vertically in the air. This is Single Leg Inverted Staff Pose.

5 Exhale, and place the hands on either side of the head. Press into the palms and straighten the arms to lift back up to Upward Facing Bow Pose. The tuck in your chin and lower your head and buttocks to the floor.

6 Once you have learned this pose, it is also possible to drop back into this posture from Headstand.

INFORMATION

GAZE Tip of nose.

BUILD-UP POSES Supported Bridge Pose, Upward Facing Bow Pose, Headstand.

COUNTER POSE Double Leg Forward Stretch.

LIGHTEN a) Do not straighten the legs fully. **b)** With bent knees, lift your heels.

EFFECT Energizing.

Advanced Bow Posture

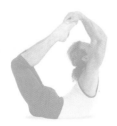

Padangustha Dhanurasana In this advanced backbending posture, the arms are like the string of a bow. This deep backbend tones the entire spine and the abdominal area and works deeply into the shoulders.

1 Lie face down on the floor and lift up to a Sphinx-like backbend. Bend the right knee to lift the foot in the air.

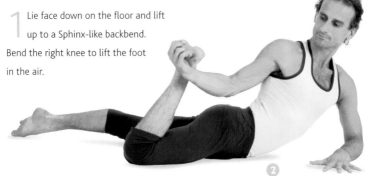

2 Supporting yourself with your left forearm, lift the right hand off the floor and reach back to the right foot. Turn the right foot out and take hold of the toes.

3 Sliding the fingers around the toes, rotate the arm outward and upward to finish with the elbow pointing up. At the same time, pull the right leg up.

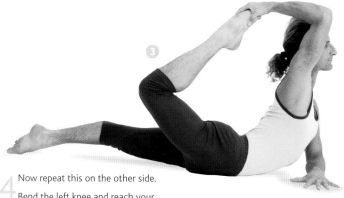

4 Now repeat this on the other side. Bend the left knee and reach your left hand back to the left foot. You will find yourself rolling forward onto your stomach. Holding firmly on to the left foot, rotate the left elbow out.

INFORMATION

GAZE Third eye.

BUILD-UP POSES Bow Pose, Crescent Moon Pose, Elbow Balance, Royal Pigeon Posture.

COUNTER POSES Downward Facing Dog Pose, Double Leg Forward Stretch, Yogic Sleep Pose.

LIGHTEN a) Hold only one foot at a time. **b)** Grasp a belt looped around the feet.

EFFECT Energizing.

5 With the weight of the body resting on your abdomen, reach the hands and feet upward. Try to straighten the arms, increasing the curve in the lower back. Stay five to ten breaths, then release the feet one at a time and come back to Cobra Pose (page 242).

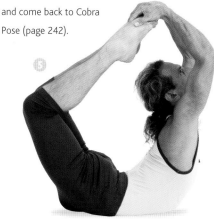

Reclining Hero Pose

Supta Virasana This pose gives the front of the thighs a fantastic stretch. It opens the pelvic abdomen and increases circulation to the abdominal organs.

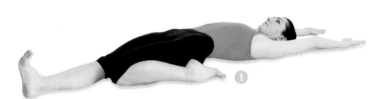

1 Warm up with Reclining Half Hero Pose first. Kneel down between your heels to sit in Hero Pose (page 120). Straighten one leg along the floor in front of you. Take the palms to the floor behind you and lean the upper body back. Lift your seat a little and extend your tailbone toward your knees to lengthen the lower back. If possible, bring the elbows to the floor so that the palms of the hands rest near the buttocks. Once again, lift your seat and reestablish the posterior tilt of the pelvis, so that the pubic bone moves closer

to your ribs. From here, keep the lower back elongated, and lie on your back. Extend the arms straight along the floor overhead or cup the elbows overhead. After holding for some time, repeat on the other side.

2 For the full Reclining Hero Pose, begin in Hero Pose with the thighbones parallel. Squeeze the inner knees toward each other as you gently contract the buttocks and lengthen the tailbone

toward the floor. Adjust your pelvis as in the preparatory position. Lift the buttocks and lengthen the lower spine, so that the sacrum can lie flat on the floor as you lay the upper body back on the floor. This will open the front of the hips and thighs deeply. Have the arms either resting beside the legs, extended overhead, or fold your forearms to cup the elbows and increase the opening in the chest.

3 Draw your floating ribs down as you slide the tailbone toward your knees. Keep as much of the spine in contact with the floor as possible as you allow the front of the body to soften and open with the breath. Keep the chin tucked in toward the chest and the back of the neck long. To come up, place the palms on or near the soles of the feet, press the forearms into the floor, inhale, and lift the chest up.

4 To practice this pose in a more restorative way, lie back on a bolster or folded blankets. To lie back in Restful Reclining Hero Pose, place the narrow edge of one to four folded blankets or a bolster against the sacrum while

INFORMATION

GAZE To infinity or eyes closed.

BUILD-UP POSES Hero Pose, Supported Bridge Pose, Camel Posture, Frog Pose.

COUNTER POSES Child Pose and Extended Child Pose, Double Leg Forward Stretch, Head Beyond the Knee Pose.

LIGHTEN a) Widen the knees apart. **b)** Just lie part way back. **c)** Practice the restorative version.

EFFECT Opening.

still seated upright, then lay the spine down along the length of the support. The back of the neck should be in one line with the spine. If the chin tilts toward the ceiling, have an additional blanket beneath the head. Rest the backs of the hands on the floor. Close the eyes and cover your body for warmth if you wish. Stay for up to ten minutes.

Pigeon Posture

Kapotasana This elegant and
challenging backbend tones the entire
spine and expands the chest. Besides
stretching the quadriceps muscles, it
targets the iliopsoas muscle deep in the
front of the thighs, which is a tight area
for many people.

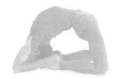

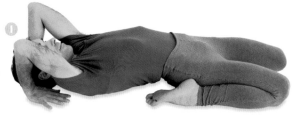

1 Lie in Reclining
Hero Pose (page
272) with the knees
together. Tuck your
tailbone under and lengthen through the
front of the legs. This will elongate the
lumbar spine and allow you to draw
the floating ribs in toward the core of
the body. Bend the elbows and place
the hands on either side of the head
with the fingers pointing toward the
feet and the elbows pointing straight
up. Take a few breaths here to
consolidate this position.

2 Wait for an inner cue to lift up.
When it comes, inhale, lift the hips
up, and straighten the arms so your head
lifts off the floor. Move the hips forward
and arch the spine back.

3 Bend the elbows a little and walk the
hands toward the feet. Then rest the
elbows on the floor, bringing them closer
together. Keep the knees close together.

INFORMATION

GAZE Tip of nose.

BUILD-UP POSES Crescent Moon Pose, Camel Posture, Upward Facing Bow Pose, Frog Pose.

COUNTER POSE Double Leg Forward Stretch.

LIGHTEN Sit in Hero Pose with a few blocks under the buttocks, then drop back slowly into a backbend supported by your arms. Then reach for the feet with the hands. Gradually learn to walk the hands in and to lift up into the full posture.

EFFECT Energizing.

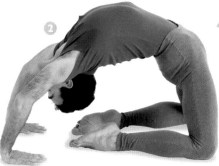

4 Exhale, lower the legs and hips down, and lie back in Reclining Hero Pose.

5 Once you have mastered this posture, it is possible to drop back into it from a kneeling position and then come back up the way you went down.

Tilt the head back and rest it on the floor between (or as close as possible to) the feet. The full posture is achieved when you can hold your heels or your ankles. Stay in the posture for as long as you can, keeping the breathing as smooth and long as possible.

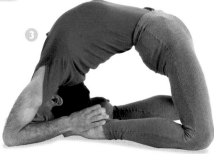

Royal Pigeon Posture

Eka Pada Rajakapotasana This
beautiful-looking posture stretches
the shoulders and vertebral column
strongly. It also helps regulate the
hormonal secretions, particularly
those from the thyroid.

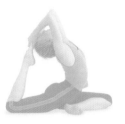

1 Perform Downward Facing Dog Pose
(page 162). Step the left leg forward
to place the foot behind the right hand
so the left knee is behind the left hand.
Slide the right leg straight back behind
you as you lower both hips close to
the floor. Stretch the toes of the
right foot back. Your buttock and
outer left thigh will be resting on the
floor. Decompress the lower

back by lifting up through the chest.
Let the front of the left thigh lengthen
as the hips descend further.
Breathe here, consolidating
your position.

2 Bend the right leg and
bring the left foot as close
as possible to the head. Turn
the foot so that the toes
are pointing to the
right. Using your
left hand for
balance, reach

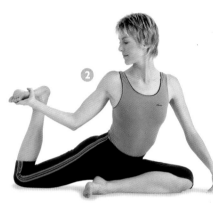

back with the right hand to take hold of the toes. Pull the right leg toward you as you rotate the arm upward and outward. Take a few breaths here.

3 Lift the left hand off the floor and reach back behind the head. Holding the raised foot with both hands, allow the head to lean back while the right foot comes forward so that the crown of the head or the forehead rests in the arch of the foot. Hold for five to ten breaths.

4 Exhale, release the hands one by one to the floor. Gently lift back into Downward Facing Dog Pose, then repeat on the other side.

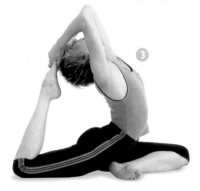

INFORMATION

GAZE Third eye.

BUILD-UP POSES Crescent Moon Pose, Frog Pose, Monkey God Posture, Pigeon Posture.

COUNTER POSES Downward Facing Dog Pose, Head Beyond the Knee Pose, Double Leg Forward Stretch.

LIGHTEN a) Sit higher by placing a rolled blanket under the perineum. **b)** Grasp a belt looped around the raised foot.

EFFECT Energizing.

Inversions

Inverted postures improve lymph and venous circulation.

They work the heart and boost the immune system.

Increased blood supply to the endocrine

glands at the throat is the reason

why inversions are considered to

be hormonal balancers.

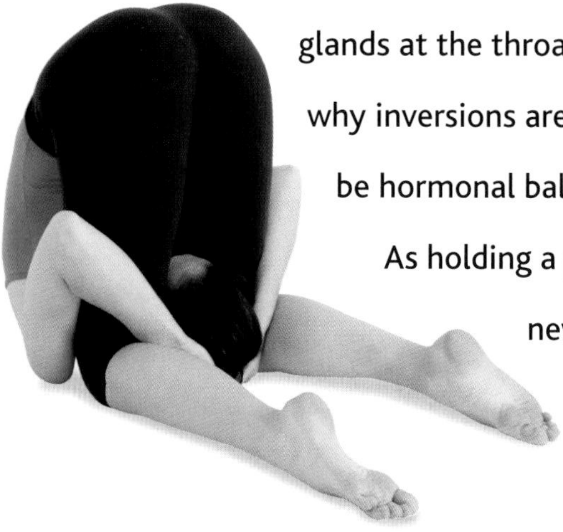

As holding a position with a whole

new relationship

to gravity demands

a certain steadiness

of body and mind, inversions are
calming poses. Inversions let us
see things from a new angle.
They lessen tiredness
and develop concentration.
As inversions quiet the mind
and settle the system down, they
are generally practiced toward the
end of an *asana* session, after your
body has been well warmed up.

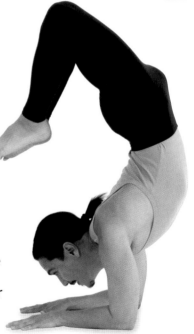

Easy Inversion

Viparita Karani This passive pose relieves congestion in the legs and is restorative for the entire nervous system. Many inversions are not beginner's poses, but this pose can be safely practiced by those new to yoga.

1 Sit with your right hip and shoulder touching a wall and have your knees bent and heels close to the buttocks.

2 Keep the hip near the wall as you lean back on your hands. Take your legs up the wall as you lower onto your elbows. Then lay your back on the floor and check your body is symmetrical.

3 With the buttocks close to the wall and legs vertical, choose your arm position. Take your palms to the abdomen or your arms out to the side. Alternatively, take the arms overhead, elbows softly bent. If you wish, tie a soft belt around the mid thighs so the legs are passively held together. Allow the shoulders to soften

INFORMATION

GAZE Close the eyes and focus on releasing with the breath.

COUNTER POSES Any standing posture.

LIGHTEN a) Bend your knees a little if it is difficult to bring your buttocks against the wall. **b)** Bend the knees down to the chest if your feet get numb.

EFFECT Restorative, calming.

CAUTION

Inversions should not be practiced by anyone who is suffering from high blood pressure or has eye problems, such as detached retina or glaucoma. They should be avoided by women during menstruation. In the case of previous neck injuries, heart problems, or pregnancy, the advice of an experienced teacher should be sought. Most inversions are not beginner's poses and it is strongly recommended that the postures are learned from an experienced teacher.

and relax into the floor. Keep the back of the neck long. Tune into the rhythm of your breath.

4 Allow the tongue to rest on the floor of the mouth and the eyeballs to sink toward the base of the skull. Stay here for up to ten minutes, breathing deeply through the whole body.

5 To vary this pose, bring the soles of the feet together and slide the heels down the wall, so the outer edges of the feet are against the wall and knees wide apart. Ⓐ Alternatively, you can let the legs fall out to a wide "V" shape to stretch the inner thighs. Ⓑ

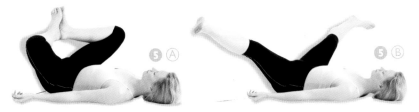

5 Ⓐ   5 Ⓑ

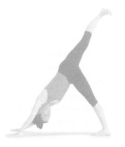

Raised Leg Downward Facing Dog Pose

Eka Pada Adho Mukha Svanasana
This pose requires stretch in the shoulders and wrists and increases flexibility in the hamstrings. It is more of an inversion than the classic pose and therefore increases the cardiac response.

1 From Downward Facing Dog Pose (page 162), bring the feet close together. Raise the left leg up, parallel to the floor. Extend the right heel closer to the floor as you press the left heel farther away. Rotate the left thigh in so the toes point straight down. Press the palms of the hands evenly into the floor and move the chest toward the thighs. Keep both shoulders an even height from the floor. Stay for five breaths, then lower the leg. Rest down if necessary. Repeat on the other side.

2 If you can raise your leg high, the following variation will give an increased stretch. From Downward Facing Dog Pose, turn your left toes out and raise the leg up toward the ceiling

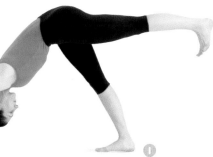

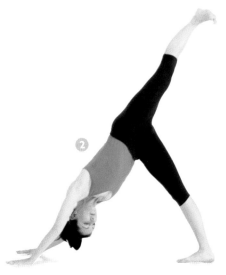

INFORMATION

GAZE Navel.

BUILD-UP POSES Downward Facing Dog Pose, Single Leg Forward Bend.

COUNTER POSE Mountain Pose.

LIGHTEN a) Don't lift the leg as high. **b)** Keep the raised knee bent. **c)** From an all fours position, raise one leg back.

EFFECT Restorative, calming.

as before but this time don't keep the shoulders level. Allow the left shoulder to move forward as the right shoulder moves back slightly, while you spiral the chest toward the left and look up from under the left upper arm.

3 Bend the left knee and let the heel fall near the buttocks. Extend the bent knee higher up and back. This will work into the abdomen and help tone the organs. Feel the whole outer edge of the left body stretch upward, from the inner

left wrist through the left underarm and along the side of the left chest to the left hip. Lower the left leg on an exhalation, then repeat on the other side.

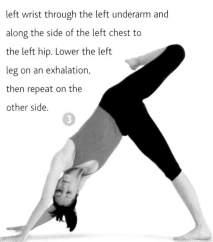

▲
Hare Pose

Sasankasana This pose gives the neck and shoulders an elongating stretch. As the intensity of the pose may be well controlled, it is a good alternative for those who are not yet ready for Headstand (page 296). The effects are rebalancing and calming.

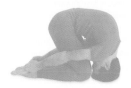

1 Start in Child Pose (page 100). Holding the heels with the hands, tuck the head in, bringing the forehead as close to the knees as possible.

2 On an inhalation, roll forward onto the crown of the head, so the chest comes away from the thighs and the buttocks lift high. On the exhalation, lower the buttocks and chest as you roll back to the starting position. Move back and forth in time to your breath a few times.

3 The final time, hold the hips high for several breaths. With hands firmly grasping heels, press your middle and upper back away to increase the space between the shoulder blades. Feel the skin stretch in the middle back as these muscles get a welcome release. Press the vertebrae of the neck away also to roll right onto the top of the head. Close the eyes and enjoy the stretch at the base of the neck and the top of the shoulders.

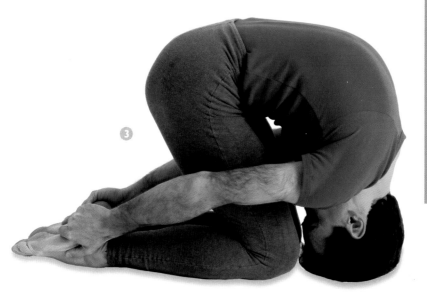

INFORMATION

GAZE Inward, eyes closed or to navel.

BUILD-UP POSE Child Pose.

COUNTER POSES Fish Pose, Corpse Pose, Neck Releases.

LIGHTEN a) Don't roll all the way onto the crown of the head. **b)** Practice with a blanket behind the knees or under the ankles if joints are stiff.
c) Place the forehead on a bolster or folded blanket if the neck is stiff.
d) Place the hands closer to the shoulders.

EFFECT Balancing.

Shoulderstand

Sarvangasana In this inverted position where the chin presses against the chest, circulation to the thyroid and parathyroid glands is increased. The endocrine glands in the brain also receive fresh blood. This pose is best practiced toward the end of your asana sequence, when you can really appreciate its deeply calming effects.

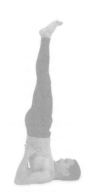

1 While experienced practitioners may be comfortable practicing on a cushioned surface, such as a soft carpet or a yoga mat, using blankets takes the strain out of the neck for beginners. Fold two or three blankets into a rectangle. Lie on your back over the neatly lined up edges of the blankets. The back of your head will be on the floor and the top of your shoulders about 2 inches (6 centimeters) away from the edge. Bend your knees up.

2 Firm your abdominal muscles to bring your legs overhead, with the knees bent. Support your back with your hands. From here, tuck your shoulders under and bring your elbows closer together. With arms outstretched, establish a good foundation for your upward lift in this pose.

3 Straighten your legs in the air. Extend up through the inner legs. Stretch out all your toes. Bring the elbows closer together. Soften the skin on your face. Enjoy the natural Warming Breath (page 332) as the chin presses toward the throat. Stay for twenty breaths or as long as you enjoy the posture. Over several months, build your time in the pose to five or ten minutes.

4 Remind yourself that you are practicing Shoulderstand, not "Neckstand." The muscles of the neck need to stay relatively soft. If they are strained tight, hinge at the hips more to fold your legs over your face and ease the pressure. This is called Half Shoulderstand

INFORMATION

GAZE Toes.

BUILD-UP POSES Easy Inversion, Supported Bridge Pose.

COUNTER POSES Fish Pose, Neck Releases, Head Beyond the Knee Pose.

LIGHTEN From Easy Inversion bend your knees and push your feet into the wall to lift your hips up. Support your lower back with your hands. If possible, take one or both legs in the air.

EFFECT Balancing.

and is the best option for many beginners. When you combine it with an awareness of the *chakras* in the line from the solar plexus to the throat, it becomes a *mudra*, Inverted Effect Seal.

5 To come down, take your legs overhead. Press your hands to the floor and lower yourself with control.

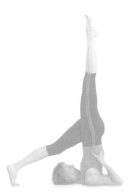

Shoulderstand Cycle

Running these variations of Shoulderstand (page 286) together makes a good sequence. If you like, include Plough Pose (page 292) and Ear Pressure Pose (page 294). Hold each variation for five to fifteen breaths.

One Leg Extended Shoulderstand
Eka Pada Sarvangasana

From Shoulderstand, keep both legs straight and lower the left leg over your head. If possible, bring the toes to the floor. Extend the right leg vertically upward, visualizing a line of energy running up the inner leg. Press away with the ball of the right foot and stretch out both sets of toes. To straighten the back more, draw in the lumbar spine, then the vertebrae of the middle back. Keep both legs straight. After five to fifteen breaths, raise the left leg and repeat on the other side.

Rotated Shoulderstand
Parsva Sarvangasana

Lower both legs over your head and to the left.
Twist your torso to the left and move your
right hand to the center of the sacrum, so
your middle finger lies in the cleft
between the buttocks. Lay your
left hand along the floor. Rotate the
torso more, then lower the left leg backward
and to the right while extending the right leg diagonally forward and to the left to create
a mid-air split. Press down through the elbows and shoulders. Firm your buttocks and
extend well through the legs all the way to the balls of the feet.

Supine Angle Shoulderstand
Supta Kona Sarvangasana

From Plough Pose (page 292), walk the feet apart to a wide
"V" shape. If your feet touch the floor, release your hands
from the lower back and move them over your head
to cup the toes. Broaden the shoulders and
spread your weight evenly across the
shoulders. To return to Shoulderstand first
take your hands to hold the back.

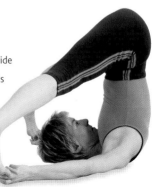

Upward Lotus Shoulderstand
Urdhva Padma Sarvangasana

In this variation the legs are interlocked in Lotus.
You will need to be able to perform Lotus Posture
(page 152). From Shoulderstand (page 286), bend the
right knee and bring the right foot into the left groin. Use
your left hand if necessary to help bring the ankle into
place. Hinge at the hips so both legs come closer to the face,
bend the left knee out to the side, and bring the left foot over
the right knee. Supporting yourself with your left hand, use
your right hand to help slide the foot down to the right
groin. After ten to fifteen breaths, release the legs, straighten
them in the air and repeat, crossing the left leg first.

Inverted Lotus Pose
Urdhva Padmasana

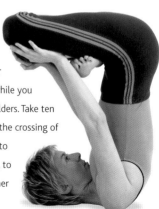

From Upward Lotus Shoulderstand, hinge at the
hips to fold your Lotus forward. Take your hands
from your lower back to your knees. Straighten your
arms and, to help balance, press up on your knees while you
press down with your legs. Broaden across the shoulders. Take ten
breaths. Each time you practice this pose, alternate the crossing of
the legs. To take this pose farther, lower your legs into
the chest. Wrap your arms around your entire Lotus, to
hug your legs in closely. Hold one wrist with the other
hand. This pose is called Embryo Pose 1.

Unsupported Shoulder Balance

Niralamba Sarvangasana

As this pose lacks the stabilizing
support of the arms, approach it
with caution if your neck needs special
care. Prepare and warm the body by practicing
Shoulderstand. Then hinge at the hips to lower
the legs slightly over your head. Release your
hands from the back and extend your arms
straight up. Working the back and abdominal
muscles well, move the legs up and back to vertical.
Extend from your shoulders to your fingertips as they
reach to the sky. Stretch out your toes. Keep the back
muscles working. Hold for ten steady breaths. Then
come back to Shoulderstand.

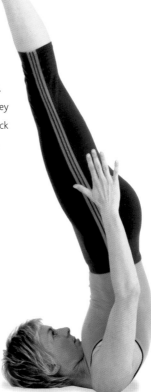

Plough Pose

Halasana This folded-over inversion is wonderfully rejuvenating to the entire nervous system. The abdominal organs are contracted and toned. The neck and shoulders are released from any habitual tension and the spine is stretched to its maximum. It is a natural pose to come to from Shoulderstand (page 286).

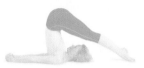

1 Lie face up on a cushioned surface, such as a soft carpet or folded blanket. Beginners may prefer to use two or three tri-folded blankets. With blankets under your back, shoulders, and elbows forming an upper level, have your head on a lower level. Lying flat, relax the shoulders away from the ears. Draw the chin in toward the chest, lengthening the back of the neck.

2 Bend your knees in toward the chest. Press the palms of the hands firmly into the floor as you extend the feet over the head, straightening the legs. If your toes don't reach the floor, then keep your palms on your lower back. Take care not to overdo it here, because this position is a very strong forward bend that also places a lot of weight on your shoulders and neck. Keep your head in line with the rest of the vertebral column.

3 Rest the toes on the floor behind the head, toes tucked under. To deepen the pose, raise the sitting bones upward as you press through the back of the legs, lengthening the hamstrings. Lift the upper chest toward the chin, bringing the spine

more to a vertical position. Bring the palms of the hands together and interlock the fingers, rolling farther onto the top of the shoulders. Press the little finger side of the hands against the floor. If possible, untuck the toes so the tops of the feet are on the floor.

4 To come down, lower your buttocks to the floor, then use your abdominal muscles to help you slowly lower the legs, keeping the back of your head on the floor. Practice some counter poses afterward to release the neck.

INFORMATION

GAZE Tip of nose.

BUILD-UP POSES Double Leg Forward Stretch, Hare Pose, Half Shoulderstand, Easy Inversion.

COUNTER POSES Revolved Abdomen Pose, Head Beyond the Knee Pose, Fish Pose, Neck Releases.

LIGHTEN a) Rest the legs (from the root of the thighs) on the seat of a chair. **b)** Bend the knees. **c)** Drape the bent arms along the floor over your head.

EFFECT Calming, restorative.

Ear Pressure Pose

Karnapidasana This is a strong forward stretch that demands a lot of flexibility in the spine while placing great pressure on the neck. Once you are comfortable. Ear Pressure Pose becomes a very nurturing pose, because you are cocooned into yourself in a soothing way.

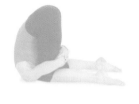

1 From Plough Pose (page 292), bend your knees to your ears. When you come into this pose from practicing Shoulderstand (page 286) on folded blankets, it is much harder to bring the shins to the floor, so you may find you need to tuck your toes under. To help lift up through the trunk, stretch your arms along the floor behind you and interlace the fingers.

2 Bring your shins and the tops of your feet to the floor so your toes point away. Wrap your arms over the backs of your knees and clasp your hands. Hold this pose for five to ten breaths before supporting the back and coming back to Plough Pose.

INFORMATION

GAZE Tip of nose.

BUILD-UP POSES Shoulderstand, Plough Pose, Double Leg Forward Stretch.

COUNTER POSES Neck Releases, Fish Pose, Head Beyond the Knee Pose.

LIGHTEN a) Rest knees on forehead or near eye sockets. **b)** Tuck the toes under. **c)** Do not bring knees to the floor. **d)** Support your back with the hands instead of wrapping them.

EFFECT Calming.

3 A more intense pose is to wrap the arms over the legs and place the hands under the head. When you combine this pose with an awareness of the solar plexus center, it becomes a *mudra*, Seal of the Noose.

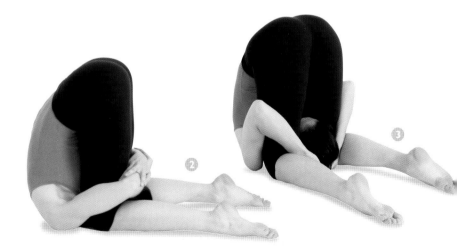

Headstand

Sirsasana Headstand has been called the king of asana, and its benefits are indeed innumerable: calming to the nervous system, nourishing to the brain cells, stimulating to the heart and circulation, balancing to the hormonal and digestive systems, and strengthening to the spirit.

1 In this classic yoga posture, the weight of the body rests on the head and arms. Since your head weighs about 9 pounds (4 kilograms) and your body considerably more, proper alignment and preparation are essential. Place a folded blanket or yoga mat in front of you. Kneel in front of your blanket. Place your forearms on the blanket, with your elbows no wider than your shoulders and form a triangle by interlacing your fingers. If you are using a wall as a safeguard from falling in the beginning, the knuckles should be 2–3 inches (6–8 centimeters) away from it.

2 When performing Headstand, it is important to lift well up from elbows to shoulders. Practice your lift by pressing

down through the elbows and moving the shoulders up toward the hips. Close the gap between the floor and the edge of your wrists. These movements should increase the distance between the shoulders and the ears and lift the head away from the floor. If you can't lift your head, you are not ready for Headstand and need to do some preparatory work to build flexibility and strength first.

3 Place the crown of the head between the wrists, with the back of the head resting against the hands. For the correct alignment in the neck, the very top of the head (not in front of or behind this area) must be in contact with the floor.

4 Tuck your toes under and straighten your knees so you are in an inverted "V" shape. Walk your feet toward the head,

INFORMATION

GAZE Tip of nose.

BUILD-UP POSES Hare Pose, Downward Facing Dog Pose, Elbow Balance.

COUNTER POSES Practice Child Pose for a few moments after coming down, Shoulderstand, Neck Releases.

LIGHTEN Get help from an experienced teacher.

EFFECT Balancing.

gradually bringing the weight of the body onto the head.

5 When the feet are as close to the head as possible, lift them off the floor (one by one, or with control, together)

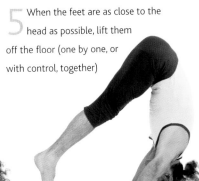

Headstand (continued)

and slowly bring the heels to the buttocks. Ground down well through the elbows and sides of the wrists. From this steady foundation, reestablish your lift upward to reduce the weight on the head and neck.

6 Once the feet are lifted, straighten the legs and stretch the heels upward. Again, press the elbows down and lift up the shoulders. If you are near a wall, it should only be used as a safeguard and not to hold you up. Your floating ribs must not jut out. If they do, lengthen the

back of the waist and tighten the abdomen to draw them in. Later you can learn to lift up with both legs straight. In any case, keep the feet together and, most importantly, do not kick up but lift up slowly, with control.

7 In the beginning stay for five breaths. Slowly build up your holding time over many months to ten minutes or more. Come down by reversing the steps you took to go up, and rest in Child Pose (page 100) for a few breaths afterward.

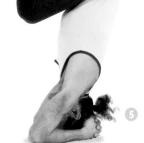

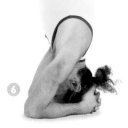

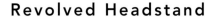

Revolved Headstand

Parsva Sirsasana In this variation of Headstand (page 296), the body is twisted so that the legs and feet are turned to the side. Headstand has a number of variations. Once you have an established practice of Headstand, link these postures together to form a flowing Headstand Cycle.

Practice Headstand. Press the elbows down strongly as you lift the shoulders away from the floor.

Exhale and turn fully to the right, taking the right hip back and the left hip forward. Keep extending the heels up. Draw the navel and floating ribs in toward the spine to avoid arching the back. With your spine as a central axis, twist as deeply to the right as possible. Keep the elbows and head stable. Exhale, come back to center, take a breath, and repeat on the other side.

A variation is to bend both knees to the heels to arrive near the buttocks, then twist, grounding down evenly through both elbows. This is called Sideways Hero Pose.

INFORMATION

GAZE Tip of nose.

BUILD-UP POSE Headstand.

COUNTER POSES Shoulderstand, Child Pose, Embryo Pose.

LIGHTEN Practice against a wall.

EFFECT Balancing.

Inverted Lotus Posture

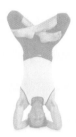

Urdhva Padmasana In this variation of Headstand (page 296), the legs are interlocked in Lotus while in Headstand. Therefore one must master Lotus Posture (page 152) before attempting it.

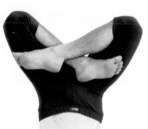

Practice Headstand and establish a steady balance. Bend the right knee and bring the right foot into the left groin. Bend the left knee and bring the left foot over the right knee. Then slide it down the right thigh to bring to into the right groin. It helps to wear smooth leggings to give the foot an easier slide along the thigh. You might also have to wiggle the left foot a little to get it in a lotus position. After ten to fifteen breaths, exhale, straighten the legs and repeat by crossing the left leg first.

INFORMATION

GAZE Tip of nose.

BUILD-UP POSES Headstand, Lotus Posture.

COUNTER POSES Child Pose, Shoulderstand.

LIGHTEN a) Practice against a wall. **b)** Have someone help you cross the legs.

EFFECT Balancing.

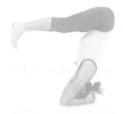

Upward Staff Posture

Urdhva Dandasana In this variation of Headstand, the legs form a 90° angle with the trunk. This requires good abdominal strength.

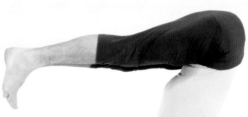

Perform Headstand. Secure your balance. Establish your foundation by pressing the elbows down as you lift the shoulders. Slowly lower the legs down to a horizontal position, keeping them straight.

Extend in a line of energy from the thighs out through the toes. As you lower, simultaneously move the hips back to maintain your balance. Keep the knees straight. Stay for five to ten breaths, then return to Headstand with straight legs.

INFORMATION

GAZE Tip of nose.

BUILD-UP POSES Headstand, Boat Pose.

COUNTER POSES Child Pose, Shoulderstand, Plough Pose.

LIGHTEN a) Lower the legs just a little. **b)** Rest your feet on a chair.

EFFECT Strengthening.

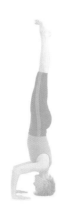

▲ Tripod Pose

Salamba Sirsasana In this variation of Headstand (page 296), the weight is borne mostly by the head, with the hands used to balance. Alignment of the head with the spine is very important. This pose is often used as an entry posture for some arm balances such One Legged Sage Balance 1 and 2 (pages 228 and 232).

1 In Tripod Pose, a little padding (such as a folded blanket) is useful. While padding helps protect the head, don't overdo it as there needs to be some firmness to stabilize your foundation and protect the head from wobbling. Kneel in front of your folded blanket. Place the crown of your head on the blanket and place your hands flat on the floor, shoulder width apart. Your fingers should point forward. Keep your elbows above the hands—don't let the elbows splay apart.

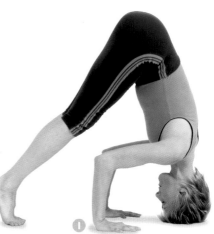

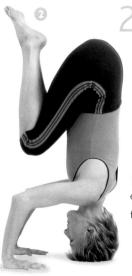

2 Tuck your toes under, straighten your knees, and walk the feet toward the head, gradually bringing the weight of the body onto the head. Inhale and press the palms evenly into the floor. Bend the knees and lift the feet off the floor.

3 Lift up into a full headstand with the feet together. As you become more experienced you can lift up with straight legs. Keep the elbows in and press down through the mounds of the thumbs. Lift the shoulder blades and shoulders up away from the floor. Stretch the feet up and draw the floating ribs in, keeping the body very straight, as in Mountain Pose (page 46). Adjust the balance with the hands as necessary.

4 Stay for five breaths. Build up over months of regular practice to five or ten minutes. Come down as you went up and rest in Child Pose (page 100) afterward.

INFORMATION

GAZE Tip of nose.

BUILD-UP POSES Headstand, Crane Posture.

COUNTER POSES Shoulderstand, Neck Releases, Child Pose, Corpse Pose.

LIGHTEN a) Practice near a wall. **b)** Get help from a knowledgeable teacher.

EFFECT Calming.

Full Arm Balance

Adho Mukha Vrksasana This posture resembles a gymnast's handstand, which commonly presents a mental challenge to adults. It asks us to overcome our fear of the unknown as we kick up into the sky. Besides requiring the mental focus to maintain balance, it develops strength in the shoulders, arms, and wrists.

1 Perform Downward Facing Dog Pose (page 162) with your hands placed 6 inches (15 centimeters) away from the wall. If the fingers are closer than this, it becomes more of a challenge to kick the legs up to vertical. Have your palms shoulder width apart, with the middle fingers pointing toward the wall. Make sure that the hands are in a symmetrical position. Walk forward until your shoulders are exactly over your fingertips. You will be on tiptoe and it will feel as though the natural progression from here is to kick up.

2 Decide which will be your dominant, "kicking" leg. Bend the other leg up, the heel near your buttock.

3 Bend your supporting leg and on an inhalation, kick it up as your other leg swings up, reaching for the wall with the heel. Remember to let your hips lift up too. Aim for a feeling

INFORMATION

GAZE Tip of nose.

BUILD-UP POSES Downward Facing Dog Pose, Raised Leg Downward Facing Dog Pose, Headstand.

COUNTER POSES Child Pose, Embryo Pose, Wrist Releases.

LIGHTEN Place a pile of blocks between the hands and rest the head onto them.

EFFECT Balancing.

of floating up the legs—visualize a ballet dancer hovering in mid-air. Bring the feet together and stretch the heels up.

4 Once you are up, remember to breathe. Grip the floor with the fingers. Let your fingertips become white. Straighten your arms well and look at a fixed point between or a little forward of the hands. As you delicately move the heels away from the wall, lengthen the back to draw in the floating ribs and free balance. Stay for five to ten breaths.

5 Once you are confident going up with one leg at a time, learn to kick up with both legs. This requires a confident, powerful kick and considerable abdominal strength. The sequence of movements is to first have your shoulders over your fingertips. When you kick up, bend your knees in, thighs close to your torso. Your hips will come into line above your shoulders. Straighten the legs up.

6 Gradually learn to balance without the wall, and then try the posture away from the wall.

Elbow Balance

Pincha Mayurasana This posture, which requires flexibility, works the shoulders strongly. In this posture, the weight of the body rests entirely on the elbows and forearms. It develops strength in the shoulders and arms and also stretches the abdomen.

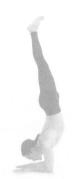

1 Place a folded blanket or yoga mat in front of you. In the beginning, practice near a wall. Kneel in front of your blanket. Place your forearms on the blanket with your elbows shoulder width apart, the forearms parallel, and the palms flat on the floor.

2 Tuck your toes under and straighten your knees so you are in an inverted "V" shape.

Your thumbs may have slid closer together, so if necessary, readjust them to bring your forearms back to parallel.

3 Walk your feet toward the arms, gradually bringing the weight of the body onto the elbows, then swing the legs up one by one, keeping them straight. Bring the feet together, straighten the legs and stretch the heels

INFORMATION

GAZE Tip of nose.

BUILD-UP POSES Headstand (Pigeon Posture for Scorpion Posture).

COUNTER POSES Child Pose, Shoulderstand, Restful Deep Forward Fold.

LIGHTEN a) Place a wooden block between the wrists to keep them apart. **b)** Practice near a wall. For Scorpion Posture, walk the feet down the wall toward the head.

EFFECT Balancing.

4 Once you have a well established Elbow Balance, you might proceed to Scorpion Posture. This resembles a scorpion ready to sting. As an advanced inverted posture with a strong backbend, it is energizing and strengthening.

5 From Elbow Balance, press the wrists down. Straighten the body up and take a few breaths. Exhale, bend the knees, lift the head, and tilt it back. Curve the spine and slowly lower the feet until the soles rest on or near the crown of the head. Keep the knees as close together as possible. Lift the chest up away from the shoulders. This is Scorpion Posture.

upward. If you are practicing against a wall, take the feet away from it. With your face toward the floor, press the elbows down and lift up through the shoulders. Keep the upper arms perpendicular to the floor. Bring your spine more to vertical. To prevent the floating ribs from jutting out excessively, lengthen the back of the waist and tighten the abdomen. Stay for five to ten breaths, then come down as you went up.

6 Stay for five to ten breaths, then either lift back up to your starting posture, or else straighten the legs a little to drop over into Upward Facing Bow Pose (page 266). From this position either release down to lie on the floor, or, if you are an advanced practitioner, stand up in Mountain Pose (page 46).

Relaxation

Yoga relaxation is time for your body to integrate the

effects of your practice. During this time for rest,

the *prana* activated by posture practice can be used

for healing and energizing the system. This is why yoga

practitioners know that, when you are tired during the

day, a period of yoga relaxation is a better investment

than taking a daytime nap.

You come out of yoga relaxation revived and refreshed with your energy boosted. And the more you practice, the better you get!

In keeping with the normal pulsatory rhythm of life, it is natural to rest after working. While you progressively let go of tension in the body, mind, and emotional heart you learn to access a deep inner peace. There is no more gripping and grasping. There is no need to hold on. Relearn how to let go.

Corpse Pose

Savasana Lying on the floor with your eyes closed allows your body to completely relax. At first, this pose can be surprisingly difficult, because we wriggle around restlessly with very busy minds distracting us from the peace available deep within our resting body. With practice, the mind and body settle down more easily.

1 Lie down on the floor with the legs stretched out, arms with hands palms up beside the body, and eyes closed. Lift the buttocks slightly off the floor, lengthening the lower back so that the sacrum is flat on the floor, and then let the spine extend toward the crown of the head.

2 Extend the legs, pushing the heels away, and then allow the legs to relax completely, feet flopping out to the sides.

3 Allow the shoulders to soften and melt into the floor. Tuck the chin in toward the throat so the back of the neck is long.

4 Unclench the back teeth and separate the lips slightly. Allow the tongue to detach from the roof of the mouth and float in the middle of the mouth, behind the lower teeth.

5 Imagine the eyeballs sinking back toward the base of the skull. Let the skin on the forehead smooth out. Let the tension release from around the eyes so it feels as if all the tiny lines around the eyes ease away.

6 Bring your attention to the breath and allow it to enter and leave the body freely through the nostrils. Imagine your whole body breathing from the crown of your head to the tips of your toes.

7 As the breath deepens, allow the body to soften and sink into the floor. It is as if you soften and relax from the outside in. Melt into the deepest layers of the body where everything is fluid. In Corpse Pose there is more than just a deep letting go; there is a sense of expansiveness too.

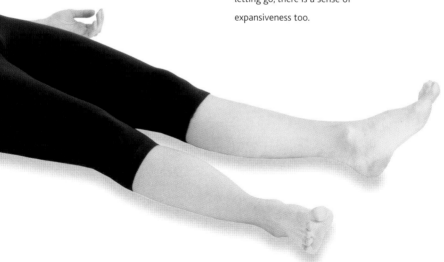

Relaxation Within Your Practice

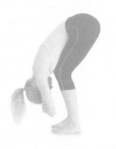

The following poses are helpful when you need to rest during your practice. The restorative poses from page 350 require a little more in the way of set up, but are great to use toward the beginning or end of your practice.

When you encounter a new posture, it can be a real challenge. It feels as if it demands all you can give and there is not a lot of room left for any relaxation. If a posture is 95 percent effort and just 5 percent release your practice might feel rather tight and constrained. However, as you become more comfortable in a pose, you'll find that it becomes less all-consuming. You will be able to hold a strong pose physically, yet still have room left to bring an element of self-nurturing to the posture. Your work to release ratio will slide to 80:20, then 70:30 and so on.

As this happens, a posture becomes steady (*stira*) and comfortable (*sukha*). Since steadiness and comfort develop with regular practice, your practice will become more rewarding as you experience more joyful freedom.

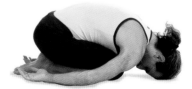

Child Pose, page 100, and its variations
Extended Child Pose, page 102

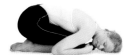

Restful Deep Forward Fold Uttanasana

This gives a break during standing postures. Modify the full Deep Forward Fold (page 68), by taking your feet hip width apart and bending your knees to rest your chest on or near the thighs. Let your arms dangle or fold them so you don't need to grip with your hands. Let the head hang down like a rag doll's. Feel your face soften and let go so much that even your cheeks droop.

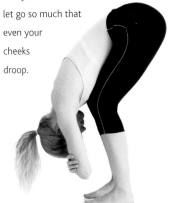

Restful Double Leg Forward Stretch

Rather than keeping the legs straight, bend them enough to rest your ribs on your thighs. Let your head drop, perhaps resting your face down between the knees. Find the most released position for your arms. Allow yourself to feel very supported.

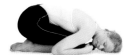

Embryo Pose, page 103

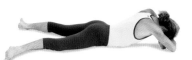

Crocodile Pose, page 246

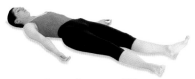

Corpse Pose, page 310

Pranayama

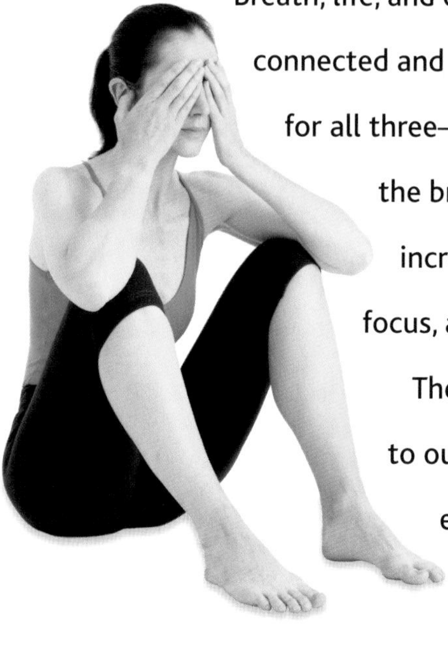

Breath, life, and energy are intrinsically

connected and yogis have a single word

for all three—*prana*. *Pranayama*, where

the breath is controlled,

increases vitality and mental

focus, and expands consciousness.

The breath acts as a bridge

to our nervous system and by

exploring *pranayama*

practices we can observe

how deeply it is connected
to the mind. Just as our breathing
alters depending on our mood,
our psychological state
can be altered by
changes in our breath.
Conscious breathing brings oxygen
and energy to the cells and enhances all cellular
processes. It's a fantastic source of energy. It's simple:
when we breathe better, we feel better.

Equal Breath

Sama Vritti Pranayama This exercise helps you release stress and come back to base. It develops a good awareness of the breath and, by fully involving the mind, it is a good concentration exercise. It feels balancing to the mind and is good when you are anxious or have trouble sleeping. It can be practiced in many places.

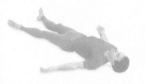

1 Lie or sit comfortably and first become aware of your natural, normal breath. After a little time, incorporate a mental count. Make your inhalation and exhalation each four beats long and continue this for five to eight rounds.

2 Next, increase the length of your inhalation and exhalation to five beats. After five or so rounds, lengthen it to six beats. Check in with how your body and mind feel. It may be that you have begun to hold tension in certain places; keep your body relaxed.

3 Lengthen your inhalation and exhalation to a count of seven each. Once again sweep over your body to be sure that no tension has accumulated. Check that the skin on your forehead is relaxed and your jaw muscles are soft.

4 After five or ten rounds, increase your count to eight beats. If your feel this lengthened breathing is causing stress, drop the count back to a number that gives you an elongated breath, yet doesn't create tension. Any force anywhere will only be counterproductive.

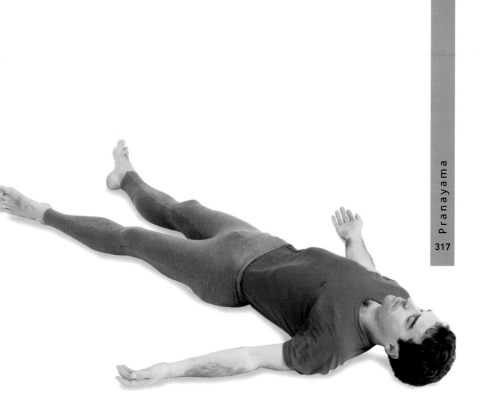

5 If you are still feeling comfortable, bring your count to nine beats. Relax the skin on your face. Relax your tongue. After some time, you may like to bring the count to ten beats. Whatever the final number, continue with this long, even breathing for several rounds. Then drop the counting and breathe naturally for ten rounds. Observe how it feels to be in your body right now. How does your mind feel? How does your emotional heart feel? More than likely you feel more relaxed than when you started. When it's time to end the practice, set your intention to keep a thread of connection to this relaxation as you continue with your day.

Humming Bee Breath

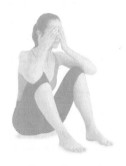

Bhramari Listening inwardly to the sound of our own breath is deeply restorative. This practice calms the emotions. It relieves anger or anxiety because it reconnects us to the nurturing rhythmic pulsation within our own being. Regular practice instantly increases our sense of well-being.

1 Choose any comfortable sitting posture such as kneeling, Easy Seated Pose (page 106), Perfect Pose (page 112), Lotus Posture (page 152), or sit in a chair. You could sit on the floor and bend your knees up in front of you. Rest your elbows on your knees in front of you to close the small flaps on the front of the ears with the tips of the index fingers. Let the spine float taller, and allow the heart center to feel open without jutting the chest up and out in an artificial way. Keep a good degree of relaxation in the shoulders, neck, and face throughout.

2 Close the eyes and bring your attention inward to the belly, the heart, the throat, and then the head. Inhale slowly to a comfortable fullness. When you come to exhale make a humming sound in the palate of the mouth. This is one round. Repeat for ten rounds or continue for several minutes.

3 Since your exhalation is now considerably lengthened, it is important to inhale unhurriedly. Don't rush into the next exhalation but take your time as you slowly fill the lungs with air.

4 Move your awareness just to the humming sound. You may like to experiment with different pitches until you find one that feels pleasurable. Feel the vibration of the sound ripple through the brain. Observe the vibrations in the face, throat, chest, and the rest of the body.

INFORMATION

GAZE Eyes closed.

BUILD-UP PRACTICE It's lovely to practice after yoga *asanas*.

AFTER THE PRACTICE Finish with seated meditation or Corpse Pose.

LIGHTEN a) Make sure your inhalations stay nice and long. **b)** Take a break if you become dizzy or light-headed.

EFFECT Soothing.

5 Sit quietly when you are finished. Keep your eyes closed. You may observe the sensations of the sound vibration pulsing through your body for some time. Don't move a muscle! The stiller you sit, the deeper your powers of observation.

Alternate Nostril Breathing

Nadi-Sodhana This practice purifies the energy channels (nadis) and balances the flow of energy between the left and right sides of the body. It is especially beneficial when you need to re-center yourself and is useful in leading you into meditation.

1 Sit in a position that gives you a straight back and is easy for you to maintain. Allow the back of the left hand to rest on top of the left knee, with the arm extended. Touch left thumb to index finger in Chin Mudra (page 334).

2 Bend the right arm and, keeping the elbow at shoulder height, bring the tip of the right thumb to rest on the bridge of the nose, just above the right nostril.

3 Have the tip of the right ring finger rest on the bridge of the nose, just

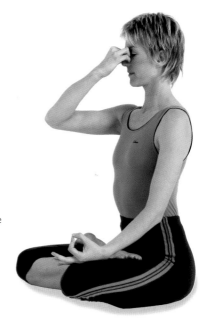

above the left nostril. The little finger lies along the ring finger. Place the index and middle fingers at the eyebrow center. This is called Nose Mudra.

4 Press the right nostril lightly shut with the thumb and inhale through the left nostril. At the end of the inhalation, close the left nostril with the ring finger and release the thumb, exhaling through the right nostril. This is one round.

5 Continue for seven to twelve rounds. If you like, use the thumb of your left hand to count the rounds against each segment of the fingers of the left hand. Bring the tip of the thumb to the tip of the index finger, then work down to the base of the finger. Move to the middle finger and so on, until the twelfth round takes you to the base of the little finger.

6 As you become accustomed to this practice, you may like to do two more cycles of twelve rounds, resting the hand down and breathing naturally in between each cycle.

7 Once this technique is comfortable, gradually lengthen the breath. Silently start counting the lengths of the inhalation and the exhalation. Make them even in length. Once they are even, increase the count by one beat and continue for a few rounds. If you still feel relaxed, increase it by one more beat. As long as the breath remains smooth and even, add one more beat. If you notice any change or disturbance in the breathing, return to a lower count.

8 During the practice, do not allow the right elbow to drag the upper body forward or take the head off center. Have the eyes closed, so it is easy to focus on the breath. When you have finished the practice, return the right hand to the right knee. Stay with your eyes closed with your normal, natural breathing for as long as you like, enjoying the sensation of inner spaciousness and serenity this practice can give you.

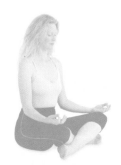

Warming Breath

Ujjayi Pranayama Use this breathing throughout your asana practice. Ujjayi means "victorious" or "expanding." In this pranayama, the breath is kept high up in the chest, rather than being allowed down into the abdomen. The chest is therefore puffed up, hence the name.

Another key characteristic of the Warming Breath is the soft sound produced by the air in the throat, and it is possible that *Ujjayi* comes from the word *Ujjapi*, which means "pronounced aloud." This sound is produced by partially closing the glottis so that a soft hissing noise is heard during inhalation and exhalation. This noise is felt as a slight contraction of the throat and helps regulate the flow of air. In Warming Breath, as in most other forms of *pranayama*, the mouth is kept closed and breathing is done only through the nose.

This *pranayama* is very energizing, and for this reason, it is best done in conjunction with Abdominal Lock (page 338) and Root Locks (page 340) (*bandhas*). The use of the *bandhas* contains the energy produced by the Warming Breath. The combination of *bandhas* and Warming Breath gives a new dimension to *asana* practice.

1 Sit on the floor in any comfortable posture in which the back can be kept straight. Keep the chin parallel to the floor, so the head is balanced, neither

tilting forward nor back. Relax your shoulders. Close your eyes. Throughout the practice, keep the attention on the throat, chest, and abdomen, without letting your thoughts stray.

2 Exhale fully. Slightly contract the perineal muscles. This is Root Lock (page 340). Before the next inhalation, direct your attention to the abdominal area and activate the abdominal muscles, slightly pulling the navel toward the spine. This is Abdominal Lock (page 338).

3 Inhale slowly and deeply through both nostrils, keeping the abdomen still. Close the glottis partially (as if swallowing) to produce an audible hissing sound. However, this sound should be soft and the breath should be relaxed. The breathing should never be strained, but only controlled. Since the abdomen is slightly contracted, it cannot push out and so the air fills the chest, which expands with the inhalation. Fill the lungs up slowly as you ensure the area between the navel and the pubis stays still. It may help to keep one hand on the abdomen to check its movements.

Then slowly exhale, keeping the throat constricted in the same way to produce this ocean-like sound. Again, keep the lower abdomen still. This constitutes one round.

4 It may be difficult in the beginning to produce the characteristic *Ujjayi* sound. This will come with practice. Remember that the most important part of the *Ujjayi* breath is the control of the abdomen and the smoothness of the flow of air.

5 When learning this technique, only do a few rounds at a time, taking a few normal breaths in between if necessary. Then gradually increase the number of rounds to fifteen as you become more comfortable with this practice.

Breathing Against the Flow

Viloma Pranayama This exercise develops conscious breathing and the ability to use the lungs fully. It is revitalizing. As you fill the lungs in three sections, visualize filling a glass with water. First the bottom part fills, then the middle, and then it fills up to the brim.

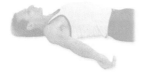

Inhale in Stages

1 Sit or lie in a comfortable position. In your mind divide the lungs into three parts. Inhale about one third of your capacity, mentally directing the air to fill the bottom third of the lungs—your abdomen will lift as you will fill up from the lowest ribs to a third of the way up the ribcage. Pause for two or three seconds.

2 Next, inhale to fill the middle third of the lungs. As you do this, mentally direct the air to the middle section of the chest, including into the side ribs and back of the torso. Your breastbone will start to lift. Pause for a couple of seconds—the air will spread through the lungs during each pause.

3 Now inhale to fill the top third of the lungs. Let your breastbone lift high as you completely fill the lungs. The tips of the lungs are located above the collarbone, so fill up under the collarbone too. It is important that you feel full to the brim, yet in a way that doesn't create stress in your system. Take any strain out of your throat area. Check that your head doesn't feel tight. To get the benefits of this

exercise, you need to feel very easy and relaxed. Once you are full to the brim, pause for a couple of seconds.

4 Now release the air in one long, smooth exhalation. Take a few recovery breaths, then repeat twice more.

Exhale in Stages

1 Come back to your natural breath. Check over your body and mind and let your tension float away.

2 Inhale in one long, steady flow. Once the lungs are completely filled, pause for a few seconds.

3 Now exhale air out of the bottom third of your lungs without tightening the abdominal muscles. As the abdomen drops, reinforce the rib cage and keep it lifted. Pause for a few seconds.

4 With awareness of the mid-section of the lungs, partially exhale for stage two, yet keep your breastbone lifted. Keep the exhalation very smooth. Pause here without inhaling any air.

5 Now exhale completely. When the lungs are nearly empty, release your lifting action on the breastbone. Patiently let the rest of the air flow out of the lungs. Once the lungs have unhurriedly emptied, pause for two or three seconds, maintaining complete stillness.

6 When your lungs call for air, inhale in one long, smooth breath to let the lungs fill deeply. Rest the lungs with a few normal breaths before repeating twice more. Rest in Corpse Pose (page 310).

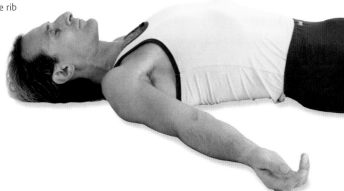

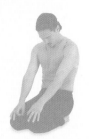

Bellows Breath

Bhastrika This pranayama draws air forcibly in and out of the lungs, fanning the flame of the gastric fire and burning the apana (accumulated waste matter) in the large intestines of the lower abdomen.

1 Blow your nose or practice Saline Nasal Irrigation (page 346) before you begin. Then sit in any comfortable position where your back is erect. Press the sitting bones down a little to allow your spine to float upward. Let the back of the neck lengthen.

2 In a quick burst, inhale sharply through the nostrils, then tighten the abdomen to exhale rapidly. This is one complete round of Bellows Breath.

3 The breath will be heard passing through the nostrils and will be similar to the sound of pumping up a bicycle tire with a hand pump. Complete ten to twenty rounds of inhalation and exhalation, expanding and contracting the abdominal muscles quickly and rhythmically on the inhalation and exhalation.

4 When you have finished, take a comfortably full inhalation. Apply Chin Lock (page 340) and Root Lock (page 340), which will contain the *prana* within, and retain the breath for thirty seconds. Then release the *bandhas* and exhale. Take several natural, easy recovery breaths. Repeat two more cycles of ten to twenty breaths. Once you are finished, lie down and rest in Corpse Pose (page 310).

5 A gentler form of Bellows Breath is Skull Shining Breath (*Kaphabla bhati*). It is considered a *kriya*, one of the cleansing techniques of Hatha yoga. The exhalation is rapid, just as in Bellows Breath. Once the lungs have been forcibly emptied, a vacuum is created, which means fresh air will naturally flow into the lungs. The inhalation of Skull Shining Breath is slow and unforced. Practice ten to thirty breaths per round and rest in between as with Bellows Breath. Over time, build up to fifty pumping exhalations.

CAUTION

When practicing Bellows Breath as a beginner, care should be taken. Start with just a few rounds and gradually build up over weeks and months. If you experience any dizziness, resume regular breathing until the breath returns to normal. Stop the practice if you experience nose bleeds. Do not practice this *pranayama* if you are pregnant or menstruating. Do not practice if you have problems with pressure in the ears or eyes.

Gazes

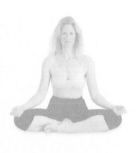

Drishtis While pranayama is generally practiced with the eyes closed, in most forms of Hatha yoga asanas are practiced with the eyes open. The eyes have an important part to play in the proper performance of any asana. Correct use of the eyes is achieved through the technique of the gazes (drishtis).

Gazes or drishtis

The *drishtis* refer to nine points or directions in which the practitioner directs his or her eyes while practicing the postures. Every posture has a corresponding *drishti*. The use of drishtis helps to develop awareness. By focusing the gaze, *drishtis* draw the mind in the proper direction for the particular *asana* that is being performed. This builds concentration and, ultimately, helps control the mind.

Much of our attention is caught up by what we see. To realize how much of our own energy is taken up by our eyes and the visual world, it can be interesting to experiment and perform some strenuous *asanas* with a blindfold. Without any visual information to process, our eyes "relax," thus releasing energy that then becomes available to the posture. In turn, blindfolded, it can become easier to hold an *asana* for longer periods (as long as we do not need to rely on visual information to hold the posture, such as in balancing postures). When our sight becomes caught up with the external, visual world while practicing yoga—the person opposite us, a chipped fingernail, what's happening outside the window—it is a sign of distraction and lack of internal focus or concentration.

The simple act of looking in a particular direction allows our energy to be focused in this particular direction. Wandering eyes distract the mind from the mind-body-spirit union that takes place during yoga practice. The single-pointed focus of the eyes helps increase mindfulness and encourages the internal focusing of the attention, rather than an external wandering. By using a particular *drishti*, it is possible to gain an internal focus and calm, while still allowing the eyes to remain open. In this respect, a posture's *drishti* is essential to the understanding of the *asana* itself, for without its respective *drishti*, a posture cannot be complete.

The *drishtis* also contain an anatomical aspect. For example, we gaze at the toes in most seated forward bends. This encourages us to lengthen the front of the body more than we would if we were looking to our navel, which would tend to cause a rounding of the back. The gaze should remain soft and light, as if detached, or as if you were looking *through* the object of your gaze. The action of gazing must not be an imposition from the mind to the eyes, for *drishtis* are meant to help release tension, not to create it. For this reason, let your practice of gazing develop over time.

INFORMATION

There are nine *drishtis*:

1. The tip of the nose

2. The thumbs

3. The third eye

4. The navel

5. Upward toward the sky, as if gazing to infinity

6. The hands

7. The toes

8 & 9. Far around to the left and the right side

Seals—Mudras

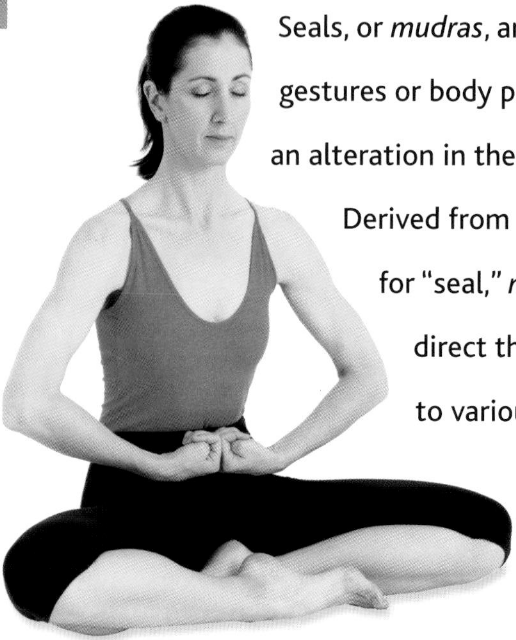

Seals, or *mudras*, are symbolic signs,

gestures or body positions that cause

an alteration in the body's vital force.

Derived from the Sanskrit word

for "seal," *mudras* allow us to

direct the pranic life force

to various parts of the body

so that these

energies may be

harnessed within.

Two of the *drishtis* are *mudras*. Gazing at the nose tip (*Agochari Mudra*) and the brow center (*Shambhavi Mudra*) are considered to calm the nervous system and increase concentration. When practiced in a certain way, some *asanas* such as Cobra Pose (page 242), Shoulderstand (page 286), and Plough Pose (page 292) become *mudras*. While Hatha yoga practice can increase *prana*, when we learn to harness this energy using *mudras* and *bandhas* (page 336), we will benefit more fully from the practice.

Meditation Mudras

These hand gestures are easily combined with yoga postures and are often used during breath work and meditation. Some *hasta mudras* are symbolic, representing a certain deity or quality. These often tie in with our understanding of the *chakra* system, Indian ayurvedic thought, Chinese acupuncture meridians, and even astrology. In general, *mudras* are considered to work through the reflex zones, by which each part of the hand is associated with a part of the body and brain.

Prayer Seal (Anjali Mudra)

Also known as *Atmanjali Mudra*, this *mudra* is often seen in India, where people use it to greet, thank, and express respect. Teachers often finish a yoga class with *Anjali mudra*, and it is a reminder to come back to your center. By regrounding yourself, you can operate from a calm, clear foundation. With this in mind, *Anjali Mudra* may be used to start and end your meditation session. The gentle pressure of the two palms against each other is believed to harmonize the left and right hemispheres of the brain. By pressing the thumbs to your breastbone you remind yourself to cultivate the qualities of the heart during your practice—try using it between each round of the Sun Salutation (pages 40 and 42).

Dhyani Mudra

This *mudra* is used for meditation and contemplation.
The left hand is placed on top of the right and tips of
the thumbs touch. Symbolically, the hands form an
empty bowl, receptive to contemplative thought.

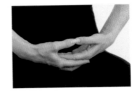

Bhairava and Bhairavi Mudras

When the right hand is on top and the thumbs are laid
down to rest one on the other, this double hand bowl is
called *Bhairava mudra*. (*Bhairava* signifies an aspect of
the god Shiva.) When the left hand is on top, thumbs
resting down, this is called *Bhairavi mudra*, named after
Shakti, the consort of Shiva.

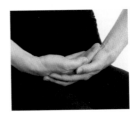

Sanmukhi Mudra—Closing of the Six Gates

This *mudra* allows our sensory organs to rest in deep silence as we let go of outer
distractions and turn our gaze inward. As the "seal of the inner source," it is also known as
Yoni mudra. Sit in meditative position. Press on the little flap in front of your
ears with your thumbs to block sound from your ears. Cover your eyes with
your index fingers, touch the sides of your nostrils with your
middle fingers, and place the ring and little fingers above and
below your lips to symbolically cover the mouth. Keeping the
elbows raised, breathe steadily in *Sanmukhi mudra* and enjoy this deep silence.
When you feel tired, lower the arms and sit in quiet stillness for meditation or
contemplation. If you wish, apply a light, equal pressure to
both nostrils while still allowing space for an even flow of air.

Prayanana Mudras— Hand Seals for Breathing Practices

Chin Mudra

Curl the thumb and first fingertip to touch each other, or alternatively, touch the index fingertip to the joint halfway down the thumb. Keep the other three fingers straight.

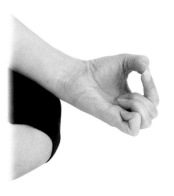

Depending on the exact position of the index finger and whether the hand is placed palm up or palm down, it may be called *Asaka Mudra*, *Jnana Mudra* or *Gyana Mudra*, Gesture of Wisdom. Here, the thumb is symbolic of the divine force and the index finger, a symbol of human consciousness. The user of this *mudra* demonstrates their intent to unite their individual oneness with the cosmic consciousness. This *mudra* alters the breath by encouraging abdominal breathing. While Chin Mudra has the palm facing up, when the palm faces down, it is called *Jnana Mudra*. In Buddhism this *mudra* is called Discussion Seal (*Vitarka Mudra*).

Chinmaya Mudra

While your index finger and thumb touch, curl the other three fingers down so their fingertips touch the palm. This *mudra*, translated as the Seal of Manifested Consciousness, encourages intercostal breathing through the expansion of the sides of the ribcage and the middle of the torso.

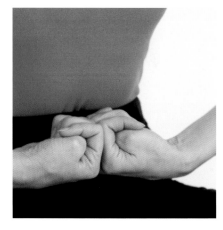

Adhi Mudra

Make a fist by first folding in the thumb and covering it with the fingers. This breathing encourages clavicular breathing through the expansion of the upper section of the lungs. Many people find the difference between no *mudra* and these "breathing *mudras*" (*Chin Mudra*, *Chinmaya Mudra* and, *Adhi Mudra*) easily noticeable when they sit quietly and carefully observe their breath.

Brahma Mudra

Make fists with the thumbs tucked in and bring the knuckles together. Rest the hands, palms up, just under the breastbone so they are level with the diaphragm. Have the little fingers touching the abdomen. As the knuckles touch, all the energy meridians of the hands are activated. This *mudra* encourages deep and full breathing. While you use it, observe each complete inhalation, which begins at the abdomen, moves up to fill the middle and side ribs and finally completely fills the very tips of the lungs right up under the collarbone. As you exhale, become aware of the gentle contracting force as the air flows out of the lungs through the nostrils.

Internal Energy Locks—Bandhas

The various techniques of Hatha yoga
have powerful effects on the production
and circulation of pranic energy in the body.
The *bandhas* are a means of controlling and
directing this energy. The word *bandha* means
"to lock" or "to restrain." It describes well the
action of *bandhas*; they lock or
restrain the *prana*. They are
essential to the advanced
practice of Hatha yoga.

Without them, the energy produced by the practice cannot be properly utilized.

All *bandhas* involve muscular contractions, but this is only one aspect of them, and the ancient yoga texts list *bandhas* among the most important Hatha yoga techniques. Practiced with *pranayama* or in isolation, the *bandhas* work with the organs and the nervous and endocrine systems. They can help to ease disorders of the reproductive and urinary systems, sexual dysfunction, back problems, and recovery after childbirth.

Abdominal Lock

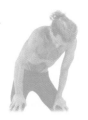

Uddyana Bandha Uddyana means "to fly upward," and the Hatha Yoga Pradipika says that through the use of this bandha, the great bird Prana is made to fly up. Unlike Root Lock, this lock channels energy in the central energy meridian (the Shushumna nadi).

Abdominal Lock is basically an inward pull of the abdominal muscles above and below the navel. When practiced on its own, it is done after a full exhalation, when the lungs are totally empty, by pulling the abdomen inward and upward.

A milder version of Abdominal Lock, can be used at the beginning of exhalation in *pranayama* practice. In *asana* practice, the contraction of the abdominal muscles stabilizes the core of the body and protects the spine. During your *asana* practice, you can start to cultivate your Abdominal Lock by controlling the lower abdominal area.

Instead of letting the lower abdominal region push out as you inhale, concentrate on keeping the area between the pubic bone and the navel drawn in toward the spine.

Practiced on its own, the full Abdominal Lock tones the abdominal organs and increases digestive powers. It is the first step toward learning Abdominal Churning (*Nauli*, page 348).

1 For full Abdominal Lock stand with the feet hip-width apart. Bend the knees slightly and bend forward. Place

your hands firmly on the thighs and round up the spine as you tuck your tailbone under.

2 Exhale fully. Hold the breath out. Lower the chin toward the chest (this is Chin Lock, page 340). This will protect the head from excess pressure.

3 Press the hands down against the thighs. Draw up your diaphragm muscle higher into your chest cavity so your abdominal area looks like it is sucking inward and upward. In the beginning, it is hard to isolate just the diaphragm muscle.

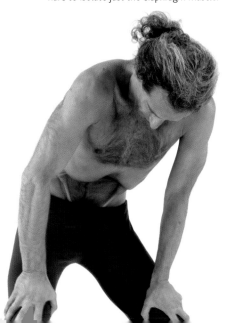

CAUTION

Abdominal Lock should only be practiced on a completely empty stomach. Do it first thing in the morning. Avoid holding the breath out for too long, which will result in strain and gasping for air. The full Abdominal Lock should not be practiced by women during menstruation or pregnancy.

With practice you will be able to differentiate and keep the abdominal wall relatively relaxed as it sucks in and up into the rib cage. (The model in this photograph is also activating Root Lock, page 340, which works the external oblique muscles and produces two visible lines that protrude from the abdomen.) Even as you hold the breath out, let your rib cage expand out as if you were breathing in. Hold for a few seconds.

4 Before you start gasping for air, release the grip on the abdomen, then slowly inhale. Stand up and take a few recovery breaths, then repeat three more times.

1. Root Lock
Mula Bandha

Root Lock is a contraction of the perineal muscles, which are located in the region between the anus and the genitals. The *Hatha Yoga Pradipika* describes it as such: "press the scrotum with the heel, contract the anus." Root Lock controls *apana*, the downward moving energy that resides in the lower abdomen, and therefore prevents *prana* from escaping downward. It is used during *asana* practice in Ashtanga Vinyasa (page 385), where it helps building internal heat. The practice of Root Lock balances the sympathetic and parasympathetic systems, improves the health of the reproductive system, and increases sexual retentive power in males. Root Lock is also said to have a powerful effect on the psychic body by triggering the awakening of the *Kundalini* energy.

Technique

To perform Root Lock, the pelvic floor between the anus and the genitals should be contracted and pulled inward and upward. In the beginning, it is difficult to discriminate between the anal sphincter, the perineal muscles, and the muscles inside the pelvic cavity. Generally people feel everything tighten up, but with practice you will learn to isolate and draw up only the perineal muscles. This is easiest on an exhalation. At first practice in a sitting position, then begin to incorporate Root Lock during forward bends and standing poses. In time, you can use this lock in all your yoga poses.

2. Chin Lock
Jalandhara Bandha

Chin Lock (pictured right) is the third of the main *bandhas*. It regulates the flow of *prana* in the area of the throat. It is said in the *Hatha Yoga Pradipika* that "Chin Lock destroys old age and death and stops the downward flow of the nectar into the fire of life." The text also states that it should be used at the end of an inhalation (*rechaka*). Indeed, Chin Lock is essential for the practice of any *pranayama* where the breath is held in (*kumbaka*). Then, by regulating the flow of *prana* to the head, it prevents headaches, dizziness, and a number of ailments of the eyes, throat, and ears that may otherwise develop.

Technique

Chin Lock is done by lowering the chin into the notch between the sides of the collarbone, thus lengthening the back of the neck. This changes the shape of the throat and slows the breathing down.

Note that the neck should bend naturally, without any tension or force.

3. The Great Lock
Maha Bandha

The Great Lock (also pictured left) is a combination of the first three *bandhas*. It can be used during *pranayama* and as a preparation for meditation.

Technique

Practice several rounds of deep breathing, such as Warming Breath (page 332). Then exhale completely. Activate Root Lock (page 340), Abdominal Lock (page 338) and Chin Lock (page 340). After several seconds, release the *bandhas*, raise the chin and inhale deeply. Repeat a few more rounds.

Yogic Cleansing Practices—Kriyas

Hatha yoga aims to allow a number of practices called *kriyas*, which are intended to help cleanse the body and balance the three bodily humors (*doshas*), ensuring good health. Two classical books on Hatha yoga, the *Hatha Yoga Pradipika* and the *Gheranda Samhita*, describe six *kriyas*. Four of these: Skull Shining Breath (page 327), Candle Gazing (page 344), Saline Nasal Irrigation (page 346), Abdominal Churning (page 348)—are described in this book and are safe to learn without a teacher. The two remaining practices require personal instruction. They are *dhauti*, the practice of cleansing the stomach with water or with a thin strip of cloth, and *vasti* (or *basti*), the practice of washing the large intestine using either water or air.

Candle Gazing

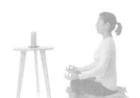

Trataka According to the Hatha Yoga Pradipika, Candle Gazing "cures diseases of the eyes and removes tiredness." It also focuses the mind, improves concentration, and is very calming. As such, it is a very good preparation for meditation. If possible, practice in a darkened room.

1 Light a candle or an oil lamp and place it on a low table, so that it will be exactly level with the eyes. Sit on the floor using a comfortable meditation posture, so there is a distance of about 1.25 yards (1 meter) between the face and the flame. Keep the back straight and the shoulders relaxed.

INFORMATION

In India, Candle Gazing is traditionally practiced using the flame of a small oil lamp, which is steadier than that of a candle. Avoid practicing in drafts. Candle Gazing can also be practiced using other objects as a focal point, such as a spiritual symbol, a drawing, or another object of significance to you (avoid mirrors). Once you have chosen an object you are happy with, don't change it but stick to using it for developing your practice.

EFFECT Cleansing for the eyes.

2 Decide in advance how long you would like to gaze at the flame. In the beginning, thirty, forty-five or, sixty seconds is realistic. Although you can't look at a clock, do your best to stick to your set time. Then this exercise will develop your equanimity and internal resilience. While initially it will be difficult to gaze at the flame without blinking for more than a few moments, this will become noticeably easier with practice. Over weeks of practice, gradually increase the gazing time from one to three minutes.

4 With eyes closed, an after-image of the flame may appear. Observe it in your mind's eye, like a focal point for your meditative mindset. When it disappears, begin your next round of gazing.

5 At the end of the third round, rub your hands together vigorously, letting the friction build lots of warmth, then cover the eyes with the cupped palms and let the eyes relax in the soothing darkness. This practice is called *palming*.

3 Gaze at the flame steadily without blinking or moving the eyes. Keep your attention totally focused on the flame. Your eyes may begin to water or you may experience some distortions of your vision. This is normal. Keep a steady mind and resist the urge to blink. When your set time is up, close the eyes gently.

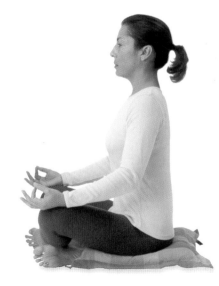

Saline Nasal Irrigation

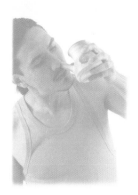

Jala Neti According to the Hatha Yoga Pradipika, Neti "cleanses the skull, makes the sight very keen, and removes diseases that are above the shoulders." It also removes mucus congestion and grit from the nasal passages. It is well worth practicing daily if you live in a dusty or polluted environment.

Saline Nasal Irrigation is performed by pouring water into one nostril and letting it run out through the other nostril. All that's needed is a dedicated *Neti* pot, available from most yoga stores and some health food stores. *Neti* pots have specially designed spouts that fit snugly inside the nostril so you can pour water down your nostrils without splashing much. If you can't find a *Neti* pot, try using a plastic container with a spout, such as those sold to hold mustard and sauces.

1 Fill the *Neti* pot with warm, salted water. Bend forward over the sink and tilt the head fully to one side. Relax, breathe through the mouth, and gently pour the salted water through the upper nostril. This is easier than you might think at first. It is a completely passive process and gravity will take care of the job. The water will flow around the septum and out through the other nostril. Do not inhale through the nose, but use your mouth. When the pot has emptied, blow your nose. Refill the pot, tilt the head the other way, and repeat for the other nostril.

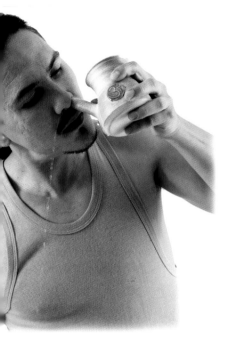

2 It is important to dry out the nasal passages thoroughly after you have finished washing the nostrils. Bend forward, close the left nostril with the fingers of the right hand, and blow your nose with a few vigorous exhalations as in Skull Shining Breath (page 327). Repeat this for the other nostril, blocking it with the thumb, then blow out both nostrils together.

INFORMATION

Make sure you put the right amount of salt in the water, so that the osmotic pressure of the water is the same at that of the body fluids. Base it on between 1 and 2 teaspoons of salt to 2 quarts (1 liter) of water. Too little or too much salt is very uncomfortable and could cause eye watering or nosebleeds. The water should be around body temperature or slightly cooler.

EFFECT Cleansing.

Abdominal Churning

Nauli According to the Hatha Yoga Pradipika, Abdominal Churning "fans the gastric fire, improves digestion, and removes all disease." Use this to start your morning yoga practice. The *kriya* strengthens the abdominal muscles and massages the abdominal organs. Its benefits cannot be underestimated.

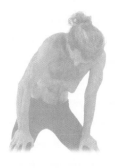

This *kriya* strengthens the abdominal muscles and massages the abdominal muscles. The benefit of Abdominal Churning to abdominal health cannot be underestimated. First master Abdominal Lock (page 338) before attempting Abdominal Churning.

1 From your Abdominal Lock, keep the abdomen drawn in and keep your chin pressing in. Press down on the hands against the thighs, and push out the abdominal recti (the two central abdominal muscles connecting the pubic bone to the sternum). Relax the recti, then the abdomen. Inhale gently and stand

up to rest. This is the first stage, which should be mastered before moving to the second stage. It often takes many practices to isolate the correct muscles, but it is really worth persevering.

2 For the second stage, press down the right hand only, pushing only the right rectus out. Sway your hips slightly to the left. Then press on the left hand, pushing only the left rectus out. Over time you will gradually learn to push the recti out left, both, right, both, left, both and so forth.

CAUTION

Abdominal Churning should only be practiced on a completely empty stomach. The best time is in the morning before breakfast. Avoid holding the breath for too long, which will result in strain and gasping for air. The inhalation should be slow, smooth and unforced. Like the full Abdominal Lock, Abdominal Churning should never be practiced by women during menstruation or pregnancy. Those with inflammatory conditions of the abdomen or other abdominal problems should consult an experienced teacher.

EFFECT Cleansing.

This will create a wave-like motion of the abdominal wall that massages the internal organs. (This exercise is sometimes referred to as the "yoga washing machine.") Practice three to five rounds, standing to rest, and taking as many recovery breaths as you need in between. Then relax.

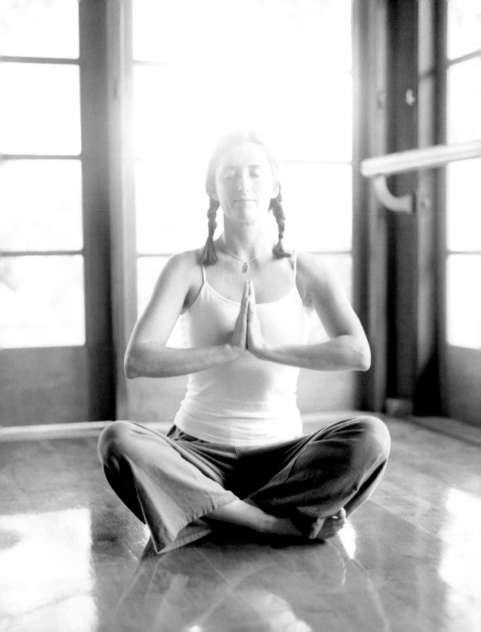

Yoga With a Special Focus

Introduction

Yoga is not a one-size-fits-all regime. The traditional Indian yoga teacher would give each student individual instructions. The individual as a whole being would be cared for and any special condition or need catered to, whether this was an agitated mind, a persistent health condition, or simply to maintain good health.

With practice, we develop an intuitive feeling for each pose. We taste the flavor of each exercise and are then able to alter the combination of our yoga ingredients to those that best suit our aims for that session.

Yoga, rooted in Eastern thought, considers each individual as more than just a mind inhabiting a body. Five dimensions or sheaths, called *koshas*, are recognized. These dimensions, from grossest to subtlest, are: First, the physical body; second, the pranic body; third, the mental and emotional body; fourth, the dimension of wisdom. Fifth, there is the spiritual bliss dimension, from where we access a sense of oneness, or transcendence. Eastern thought considers that no one dimension can ever be independent of another. An imbalance anywhere can manifest on that same plane or another. This concept of ourselves as multidimensional beings is gaining greater acceptance in the West.

Yoga is a superb holistic therapy and an excellent rebalancer. Seeking to harmonize the parts that make up all of us, yoga effectively covers all bases under the body-mind-spirit paradigm.

A combination of yogic practices will target each of the sheaths. On the physical level, you can practice *asanas* and yogic *kriyas* and maintain a good diet. *Pranayama* and *kriyas* work on the level of the vital force. The mental, emotional, and wisdom *koshas* benefit by the practice of discrimination, analysis, learning, experience, meditation, and the devotional aspects of yoga, such as chanting and turning one's thoughts to God. Feed the bliss sheath with the practice of relaxation and meditation.

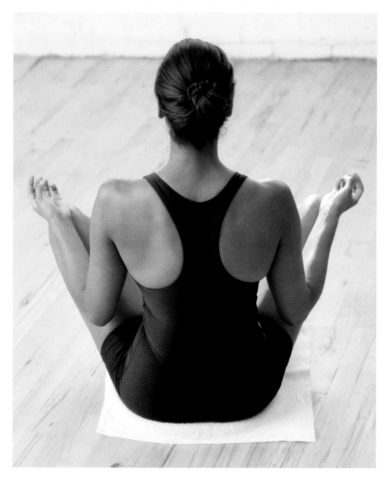

Yoga practice is made up of a combination of ingredients that can be altered depending on the aim of the session. Sometimes there are special conditions that need to be catered to.

Yoga for de-stressing

When was the last time you complained you felt stressed? For most of us that would be just hours, days or a few weeks. In our lives today we are faced with a cascade of potential stressors. A near miss crossing a busy road or just watching the latest tragedy on the news sends our adrenal glands into overtime. Living in a high adrenaline haze is hard on our bodies, unpleasant to our psyches, and tough on our emotional selves. It's no fun, so we need to find ways to counter it. Yoga helps the unwinding process when we get uptight and helps us de-stress proactively.

The *asanas* are a great channel to physically work out mental stress. Concentrating on body awareness during the practice of any *asana* gives a welcome mental break from habitually worrying about other things and is partly why people feel so refreshed after yoga. For physical and mental fatigue, the following restorative sequence of *asanas,* practiced in a slow, restful way, is helpful. These poses open the body while giving the nervous system a chance to to rest. They allow you to recharge energetically without using energy. Aside from countering stress, these postures help build energy reserves during chronic illness or menstruation, or whenever you need to rejuvenate.

In addition to the new poses shown in this section (page 356), there are other restorative *asanas* already covered that can be made part of a routine.

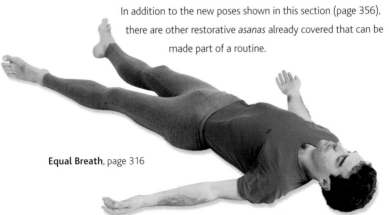

Equal Breath, page 316

Reclining Bound Angle Pose, page 136

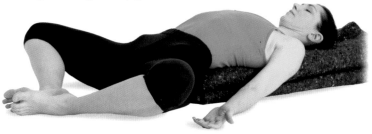

One practice routine might be: Centering with Equal Breath (page 316), Reclining Bound Angle Pose (page 136), supported Reclining Hero Pose (page 272), Child Pose (page 100) or Embryo Pose (page 103), or Restful Deep Forward Fold (page 313), Crocodile Pose (page 246), Cross Bolster Backbend (page 356), supported Plough Pose (page 292) or Easy Inversion (page 280), supported Revolved Abdomen Pose (page 190), Restorative Forward Bends (see page 357), and other supported forward bend variations (also listed on page 357). Follow with a long Corpse Pose (page 310) to counter mental and physical tension, and Alternate Nostril Breathing (page 320) or Humming Bee Breath (page 318) to calm the nervous system. Practice meditation as an all-round rebalancer.

Plough Pose, page 292

Supported Child Pose Salamba Balasana

Sit on your heels with big toes together
and knees wide apart. Bring a
bolster or stack of folded
blankets to your groin.
Lay your torso on the
support, which should
be high enough to
have your torso parallel to the floor

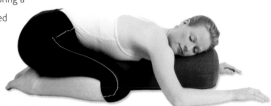

and long enough that your head is supported too. Take the arms out to the side, elbows
in line with the shoulders. Turn to rest on one cheek. Tune into the soothing way the belly
presses into the bolster on each inhalation, giving it a nurturing massage. Stay for one to
five minutes, letting all the tension drain away.

Cross Bolster Backbend Salamba Urdva Mukha
Salabhasana Sit atop two crossed bolsters or the equivalent in folded blankets.
With knees bent and feet on the floor, lie back along the bolster and bring shoulders
and head to the floor. Straighten the legs as much as is comfortable. You may even tie a
soft belt around the thighs to hold them in place. Position your hipbones as the highest

point of your arch. Rest here for two to
eight minutes. To come up,
roll off the bolsters
to one side.

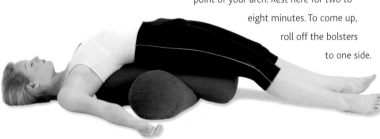

Bolster Twist Salamba Jathara Parivartanasana

Kneel with your right hip next to a bolster, feet to your left. Take one hand to either side of the bolster and rotate your torso so your breastbone is parallel to the bolster. Lay your torso along it, and bring forearms onto the floor. Turn your head to the opposite side to your legs. To increase the twist, slide the top leg along the floor away from the hips. Stay for one to six minutes, then repeat on the other side.

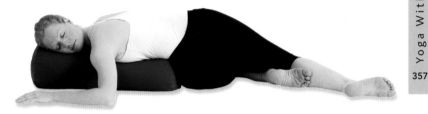

Restorative Forward Bends

You can use support in the same way for many other forward bends such as One Leg Folded Forward Bend (page 122), Head Beyond The Knee Pose (page 114), Cobbler's Pose (page 134) and Seated Angle Posture (page 130), and Seated Side Stretch Sequence (page 132). For this forward bend (*Salamba Paschimottanasana*, pictured below), sit with your legs together. Place a bolster or folded blanket on your legs and have the height so that when you fold forward your chest and cheek are fully supported on it. Find a comfortable position for the arms. If you feel too much stretch, use cushions to raise the level of your forehead.

After some time in the pose, your body will release and you'll find you can slide the support toward your feet to deepen the stretch. Hold for one to two minutes.

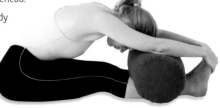

Yoga for Healing

Our internal world exists in constant interaction with our external world; we live in a state of flux. As we are ever-evolving beings, what best suits each individual changes from day to day. Consider each suggested practice as a potential ingredient in healing, but not as a set recipe. Posture suitability depends on a variety of factors, and it's a good idea to consult a yoga therapist or experienced teacher.

Special Uses of Yoga

Other recommended postures

Anxiety Conscious breathing shifts your thoughts away from your concerns and brings you right back to the present moment. Come back to your breath many times throughout the day. *Asana* practice is a great way to work stress out of your system physically and clear your head. Don't close your eyes; practice with full body awareness and use Warming Breath (page 332). After the *asana* work, release yourself during a long Corpse Pose (page 310) and practice *pranayama* and meditation every day.

Shoulderstand (page 286), Plough Pose (page 292), Equal Breath, counting breath 4 up to 10 (page 316), Humming Bee Breath (page 318), Alternate Nostril Breathing (page 320).

Arthritis Yoga may cause painful flare ups in the short term because more mobility is required from the joints. A little discomfort is acceptable in the short term because it means the joints are loosening in the long term. The trick is not to let the flare up be more than bearable and remember that your threshold will change from day to day. Practice joint limbering movements first of all. If it is difficult to hold a pose, don't stay in it for long. Instead, develop mobility in the joints by moving in and out of the pose with easy flowing movements. Use props where necessary.

Limbering exercises.

Asthma Many people have used yoga to cure their asthma. Backbends are useful because they lift and open the chest, encouraging fuller breathing. Pay particular attention not to collapse the chest in while practicing forward bends. Use Warming Breath (page 332) with your

Cat Pose (page 32), Cobra Pose (page 242), Equal Breath (with exhalation longer than inhalation, page 316), Humming Bee Breath (page 318), meditation.

Special Uses of Yoga

asana practice. *Pranayama* practices will retrain the breath and help you develop a longer exhalation.

Back Pain There are so many causes of back pain that it's best to get a correct diagnosis from a doctor and then find an experienced teacher who can advise on what approach to take. You might start with gentle standing postures and breath work. Once accustomed to this, introduce slow backbends, gentle twists, and seated forward bends. Practice abdominal strengtheners because they will help protect the back. During Corpse Pose (page 310), bend the knees or place a bolster under them. (See also Herniated [Slipped] Spinal Disc, page 361).

Wide Leg Forward Bend (page 66), Revolved Easy Pose (page 180), easy version of Boat Pose (page 178) and Revolved Abdomen Pose (page 190) with bent knees, Locust Pose (page 238), Restful Double Leg Forward Stretch (page 313), Abdominal Lock (page 338), Root Lock (page 340).

Cancer Help the body regulate itself by sticking to a low-chemical, low-stress lifestyle and choose a yoga practice that nurtures you so that you will be more naturally drawn to lifestyle choices that support a healthy *bodymind*. Choose a balanced array of *asanas*, with plenty of time for relaxation, *pranayama*, and meditation to assist in coping with physical and mental distress on the journey of life.

Shoulderstand (page 286), Plough Pose (page 292), restorative yoga. (See Yoga for de-stressing, page 354.)

Confidence Building Backbends lift the heart center and lessen introversion. Standing and balancing postures give you confidence in standing your ground. Meditation allows you to get to know yourself. Sticking to a regular, disciplined practice is in itself confidence building.

Warrior Pose I (page 60).

Constipation Stimulate peristalsis by moving through the Sun Salutations (page 40). Forward bends and twists, where the abdomen is compressed by another body part, will massage the digestive organs and encourage elimination. Inverted postures also help to get things moving. Rehydrate before and after yoga practice. Practice Skull Shining Breath (page 325), and Abdominal Churning (page 348) every morning.

Revolved Side Angle Stretch (page 82), Revolved Head to Knee Pose (page 116), Seated Half Spinal Twist (page 182), Bound Sage Pose/Twist B, C, and D (pages, 184, 198, and 200), Bow Pose (page 252), Shoulderstand (page 286), and its variations.

Depression To help stay in the present moment, keep the eyes open during *asana* practice. Involve every part of the body in every single pose and feel the bodymind come alive. Avoid long holding of forward bends because they tend to make you more introspective. Practice plenty of backbends and do practice every day, even if only a

Special Uses of Yoga

little. There are so many ways to meditate. Make sure your meditation practice really does suit you and doesn't make things worse.

Diabetes Twists and backbends tone the pancreas. Yoga *asanas* in general support the nervous system, increase circulation, and improve overall vitality.

Bound Sage Pose/Twist B, C, and D (pages 184, 198, and 200), Revolved Abdomen Pose (page 190), Bow Pose (page 252), Supported Bridge Pose (page 260).

Elderly People Although your postures might not be as extended as those in the photographs, they still carry the same benefits. Practice the limbering exercises and flow into and out of poses, rather than holding them, so that agility, strength, and flexibility develop. Practice standing balances to protect yourself from falls. Use props where necessary, such as lightly touching a wall to help with balancing. You can twist and forward bend seated in a chair, and you can even lean back over the backrest to create your own backbend. Whatever your physical state, relaxation, *pranayama*, and meditation are always possible.

Enlarged Prostate Increase vitality to the pelvic area with Reclining Bound Angle Pose (page 136), and forward bends. Easy Inversion (page 280) may also help relieve minor blockages.

Bow Pose (page 252) and other prone backbends.

Eye Fatigue Computer work demands a fixed focus at the same distance from the eyes. Look beyond your screen at regular intervals during the day. Make use of the gazing point listed for each pose (and see *Drishtis*, page 328) in all postures. Work your eyeballs in each pose, such as looking as far right as you can when twisting your torso to the right and as far up as possible when gazing to infinity in backbends. Candle Gazing (page 344) is considered to be cleansing for the eyes. There are books available on natural vision improvement that have yoga-style eye exercises.

Fatigue—Mental and Physical A gentle general practice, working each part of the body, is in order here— start with the limbering exercises. To invigorate a tired mind, Sun Salutation (page 40) gets the body moving and encourages a regular breathing rhythm to increase overall oxygenation. Backbends and inversions clear the mind.

Special Uses of Yoga

The more you can involve yourself mentally in what you are doing, the better. A twenty-minute Corpse Pose (page 310) is a better restorer during the day than taking a nap—cover your body with a shawl and lie on the floor rather than in bed so you don't fall asleep. Rest and restore physical fatigue with seated forward bends (try placing your chest on a bolster), and Corpse Pose. Re-energize with *pranayama*. If your fatigue has a sudden onset, or you can't find a cause for it, see a medical practitioner.

Fever Yoga *asanas* are best avoided when you have a fever. The *pranayama* exercises in this book can increase heat in the body, so they too should be avoided. Practice relaxation and meditation until you are over your illness and can resume *asana* practice, starting with the restorative yoga *asanas* (shown in Yoga for de-stressing, page 354).

HIV Positive Refer to the entries for Cancer and Immune Support.

Headaches—Tension See the section on Yoga for de-stressing and the entry on Neck Pain.

Herniated (Slipped) Spinal Disc Yoga can effectively manage slipped discs and disc lesions and they can heal with time and care. Forward bending should be avoided initially because the affected area of the back needs to be kept concave while bending forward. Support the area by using abdominal strengthening exercises, such as a bent leg Double Leg Raises (page 176), and practice backbends within your limits. Gradually introduce controlled twists. Flexibility in the hamstrings needs to be developed, so when it is time to introduce forward bends, begin with Reclining Hand to Toe Sequence (page 164), which keeps the back relatively stable. Allow twenty-four hours for feedback from your body before you increase the intensity of your practice. *Pranayama* and meditation practice help calm a mind troubled by chronic pain.

Hypertension Exercise dilates the blood vessels, which in turn lowers blood pressure. However, if your blood pressure is very high, it is best to keep the head above the body and

Corpse Pose (page 310), Humming Bee Breath (page 318), Alternate Nostril Breathing (page 320), Equal Breath, counting breath 4 up to 10

Special Uses of Yoga

where it is not, use Chin Lock (page 340). Practice relaxation, *pranayama*, and meditation. Take care not to hold the breath in any posture—work with Warming Breath (page 332) or circular breathing where you move straight on to the exhalation after inhaling, and vice versa. Work under the guidance of an experienced yoga teacher. Once you become adept at yoga practice, you may be able to feel more intuitively which postures are not appropriate on a given day. If stress is the cause, maintain a regular yoga practice. (See Yoga for de-stressing, page 354.)

(page 316), meditation.

Avoid: Be cautious of poses where the head is below the heart, (especially for long holds), such as Deep Forward Fold (page 68). Downward Facing Dog Pose (page 162) and the other inversions. Use Chin Lock (page 340) to protect the head from a rise in blood pressure. Be cautious of Abdominal Lock (page 338). Work with an experienced teacher.

Immune Support Regular practice of a well-rounded group of postures assists all bodily functions. After *asana* practice, take extra time for Corpse Pose (page 310) and for *pranayama*. While *asana* practice encourages health on the cellular level, Corpse Pose greatly assists healing on a deep level. *Pranayama* calms the mind and relieves the stress associated with chronic illness. Meditation opens the mind to the idea of something greater than ourselves, and many people find this supportive and healing.

Shoulderstand (page 286). Never underestimate the healing power of meditation.

Indigestion Twists, forward bends, and backbends all tone the digestive organs. Remember, yoga is best practiced on an empty stomach.

Hero Pose (page 120), Reclining (Half) Hero Pose (page 272), and Reclining Bound Angle Pose (to assist digestion). Bound Sage Pose/Twist B, C, and D (pages, 184, 198, and 200), Revolved Abdomen Pose (page 190), Bow Pose (page 252), Supported Bridge Pose (page 260), Shoulderstand (page 286). Practice Abdominal Churning (page 348) first thing in the morning (but see caution).

Avoid: Abdominal Churning (page 348), in inflammatory bowel conditions.

Insomnia Fully working the mind and body allows both to settle in deep rest more easily afterward, so fully involve your mind in your physical practice. Practice energy-raising exercises such as Sun Salutation (page 40) and backbends in the mornings. If your practice is closer to bedtime, focus on forward bends and inversions. Before bedtime practice Alternate Nostril Breathing (page 320) and meditation.

Shoulderstand (page 286), Plough Pose (page 292), Corpse Pose (page 310).

Special Uses of Yoga

Other recommended postures

Jet Lag Jet lag is a real stress on the *bodymind*, so on arrival practice restorative poses. (See Yoga for de-stressing, page 354.) Practice seated forward bends by placing a bolster or blankets under the chest to support it so the poses are more restful to the brain. In all poses, focus on slowing and steadying the breath. Inversions are considered "cooling" to the brain and help reduce congestion in the legs from long hours of sitting.

Downward Facing Dog Pose (page 162), Supported Bridge Pose (page 260), Shoulderstand (page 286), Easy Inversion (page 280), Corpse Pose (page 310).

Leg Congestion (from either standing or sitting)

The body is meant to move and the peristaltic working of the muscles around the lymphatic ducts stimulates the lymphatic system, whose job it is to clear excess fluids from the tissues. Sun Salutation B (page 42) gets the body moving. Inversions help reduce congestion in the legs from long hours of sitting. (See also Varicose Veins, page 365.)

Inverted postures such as Shoulderstand (page 286) and Easy Inversion (page 280).

Menstrual Cramps, Yoga During Menstruation

It is generally recommended that strong twists and strong backbends are not practiced during menstruation. Inverted postures may slow the flow, so they are avoided too. Forward bends are recommended during this time. Often women prefer a gentler practice during menstruation and they may enjoy some of the restorative poses. (See Yoga for de-stressing, page 354.)

Menstrual Disorders (Hormonal Imbalances)

Backbends, forward bends, twists, and Sun Salutation (page 40) increase vitality to the pelvic area. Reclining Bound Angle Pose (page 136) and Plough Pose (page 292) are key poses. By bathing the brain (and therefore its endocrine glands) in blood, inverted postures are of assistance in balancing hormones.

Bound Sage Pose/Twist B, C, and D (pages, 184, 198, and 200), Supported Bridge Pose (page 260), Locust Pose (page 238), Bow Pose (page 252), Revolved Abdomen Pose (page 190), Shoulderstand (page 286), Headstand (page 296), Corpse Pose (page 310).

Avoid: While inverted postures are of assistance in balancing hormones they should be avoided during menstruation.

Neck Pain First, get a diagnosis to find the cause. If the cause is muscular, use the limbering neck release. In twists, first look all the way behind, over the back shoulder, then turn the head to look all the way over the front shoulder. In both positions, raise one ear up to stretch that side of the neck and find the optimal releasing position for your

Special Uses of Yoga

own neck. When back-bending, keep the back of the neck long and chin tucked in a little—like a gentle Chin Lock (page 340) during postures. Where there is no risk of toppling over, practice postures with eyes closed and give your full attention to the neck—make sure you are not unwittingly overstretching it. Don't hunch the shoulders in standing poses, nor round them in forward bends. Approach Shoulderstand (page 286), Plough Pose (page 292), and Headstand (page 296) with caution. Use a pillow in Corpse Pose (page 310) if your chin juts up in the air. Throughout your entire practice, mentally visit the neck muscles, remind yourself to unhunch your shoulders, and check that the neck and shoulders feel happy.

Obesity Sun Salutation (page 40) will help to burn energy with calories. Practice plenty of standing poses, backbends, and inversions. If you think you overeat due to emotional factors, maintain a regular *asana* practice and include *pranayama* exercises and meditation to settle the nerves and emotions.

Posture Yoga works wonders to correct bad posture. Try to attend classes where there are experienced teachers who can make sure you are practicing poses with correct alignment (Iyengar yoga is a good place to start). Standing poses use the whole body in an integrated way. Choose postures to target your tighter areas, which, in a flow-on effect, tend to create less-than-perfect posture in other areas too. Shoulder opening poses and backbends help rounded backs. Use forward bends for tight hamstrings, and so on. Your daily practice can be away from the yoga mat too—it might include checking your alignment while standing in Mountain Pose at the bus stop.

Mountain Pose (page 46).

Premenstrual Tension See Menstrual Disorders, page 363.

Pregnancy Pregnant women seem to have an intuitive understanding of the essence of yoga, and many find it helps them during pregnancy and labor. The first trimester is not a safe time to begin yoga, so wait until after that. The modifications to the postures are numerous, so to fully enjoy the benefits of yoga during this special time,

Seated Angle Posture (page 130), Cobbler's Pose (page 134), Corpse Pose (page 310), soothing *pranayamas*, meditation.

Avoid: Don't begin yoga during the first twelve weeks of pregnancy. Don't practice Skull

Special Uses of Yoga

find a local prenatal yoga class. Some pointers are: Keep a "flow" feeling with your yoga at this time. Don't hold poses for a long time, but flow in and out of the postures a few times. In general, inhale upward and exhale downward, so if you keep moving and breathing in time, you are developing breath awareness that will help with labor. In every pose, make space for the blooming belly. Keep wide legs for many poses that normally have feet like Deep Forward Fold (page 68), Downward Facing Dog Pose (page 162), and seated forward bends. Enjoy all types of forward bends, but as the ligaments soften in pregnancy, take care not to overstretch them. With the twists, rather than turning your torso toward a closed space (i.e., the thigh of a bent leg), turn the other way so you are twisting your belly toward a big open space. Past a certain point, rather than lying on your abdomen for backbends, practice a flowing Supported Bridge Pose (page 260). For the relaxation, lie on your side using cushioning as a pillow and between your legs.

Stress See Yoga for de-stressing (page 354).

Varicose Veins Get clearance from your doctor and ask whether you have any existing blood clots that may be dislodged. Once you have medical clearance, all *asanas* are useful since they boost circulation. To stop varicose veins from worsening and to decrease the symptoms of existing ones, stimulate the circulation with Sun Salutation (page 40). Be sure to include the inverted postures such as Easy Inversion (page 280), Shoulderstand (page 286) or Headstand (page 296) in every practice. A wonderful practice at the end of the day is fifteen minutes of steady breathing in Easy Inversion. (See also Leg Congestion, page 363.)

Wrists and arms The computer era means we need to make sure to keep our wrists and arms healthy. Since they are integrally linked to the rest of the body, particularly the shoulders and neck, do maintain a balanced yoga practice. Yoga has had good results in a published study on carpal tunnel syndrome.

Shining Breath (page 325), Abdominal Churning (page 348), or the full Abdominal Lock (page 338). Inversions need to be done safely so there is no risk of falling. Work with an experienced teacher for guidance on this.

Practice the arm positions from Single Leg Forward Bend (page 74), Cow Posture (page 140), Eagle Pose (page 80), Downward Facing Dog Pose (page 162), and Crane Posture (page 216). Afterwards, counterpose the wrist action by using Forearm Releasing Forward Fold (page 70).

Meditation

Throughout history and in all cultures, people have sought ways to go beyond the limitations of habitual living and discover more about themselves and the nature of reality. Meditation means "to become familiar with," and is a way of exploring the inner self. In our busy lives where the senses tend to be drawn outward, meditation is a wonderful opportunity to turn inward on a journey of discovery.

People meditate for a variety of reasons. Many of us use meditation to relax and cope with stress. Meditation does help slow or still the mind and balance the emotions. People use meditation for healing. Meditation can also assist in problem solving by leading us to insights, which may range from the spiritually significant to the mundane. It can take us to higher states of awareness, peace, and clarity. Sometimes people experience visions or feelings of bliss, vitality, and an increased sensory awareness. Some have a sense of connecting with a higher aspect of themselves, or with the divine.

There are many techniques of meditation. Ask yourself what you need to achieve and find a meditation to match that goal. It's a good idea to experiment with a range of meditation techniques until you find one that resonates with you. Practices such as the Relaxing Meditation (page 369) and Five Senses Meditation

Release yourself from the expectation of needing to reach a certain point during each meditation.

(page 374) described later are great places to start. Once you have developed your ability to concentrate you might like to try the Imagery (page 371) and Sound (page 372) meditations.

While a good meditation teacher can be extremely helpful, a lot of good work can be done on your own. If you decide to find a teacher or to attend meditation classes, make sure you shop around. A great number of individuals and organizations offer training in spiritual practices and they range in quality and suitability for your unique self. Be cautious of any group that is too restrictive, controlling, or dogmatic.

Ultimately, meditation is a personal pursuit. Once you have practiced a technique as taught, feel free to experiment and adapt it to your own preferences. Avoid simply believing whatever you read or are told—test it against your own experience and intuition and come to know the truth of the matter for yourself.

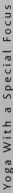

Over time sticking to a set hand seal conditions your mind to settle ready for meditation.

Establishing a regular habit of meditation works best and is easiest to maintain in the long run. Find a time that fits into your routine, whether day or night. A daily practice session of fifteen to thirty minutes works beautifully. If you find this difficult to achieve, start with five to ten minutes daily. Many people find that over time their meditation time starts to extend naturally.

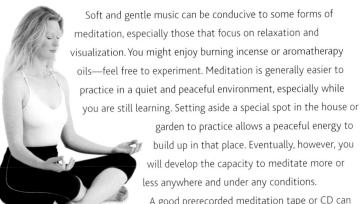

Soft and gentle music can be conducive to some forms of meditation, especially those that focus on relaxation and visualization. You might enjoy burning incense or aromatherapy oils—feel free to experiment. Meditation is generally easier to practice in a quiet and peaceful environment, especially while you are still learning. Setting aside a special spot in the house or garden to practice allows a peaceful energy to build up in that place. Eventually, however, you will develop the capacity to meditate more or less anywhere and under any conditions.

A good prerecorded meditation tape or CD can make a big difference, especially in the initial stages of your meditation practice. Alternatively, you may choose to record your own, using the following exercises as a basis. Keeping a personal journal of discoveries and experiences will enhance your progress in meditation. There is no "right" or "wrong"—whatever you experience is just fine. Keep an open, curious mind as to what you actually are experiencing. You may need to persevere before the benefits become obvious. Be patient and accept that this is a valuable part of the process. The rewards of regular, persistent, intelligent meditation practice are two-fold. They happen not just some time in the distant future, but along the path as well.

Learn to sit comfortably erect and still on the floor. If you wish, you can use cushions.

Meditation Positions

The most important thing about choosing a posture is to find one that is comfortable. Ideally, this posture will allow your spine to be relatively straight without undue tension. Your practice of yoga postures will be of great help in learning to sit comfortably erect and still.

Corpse Pose (page 310) is a great position for meditation techniques that are based around relaxation. You may like to put a small cushion under your head or larger one under your knees.

Full Lotus Posture (page 152) is a classic meditation position, but generally it is too strong for Westerners' bodies. Half Lotus Pose (page 152) works for some, and many people find sitting cross-legged in Easy Seated Pose (page 106), Perfect Pose (page 112) or kneeling are more realistic alternatives for everyday use. Be sure to use enough cushions so that your hip joints are higher than your bent knees. This will allow your back to come more to vertical.

Sitting upright in a chair is another good position for meditation. The most comfortable height is where your knees and hips form right angles. Ensure your feet can easily reach the floor—you can place them on telephone directories if necessary.

Relaxing Meditation—Deep Physical, Mental, and Emotional Relaxation

The ability to relax on physical, emotional, and mental levels is an essential skill for maintaining health and well-being and is an important starting point for those new to meditation. Since it enhances all other forms of meditation, this practice is useful for more experienced meditators. Record the following sequence onto a tape, or ask a friend to record it for you. Allow fifteen to twenty minutes.

The position of the feet in this advanced meditation position requires great flexibility.

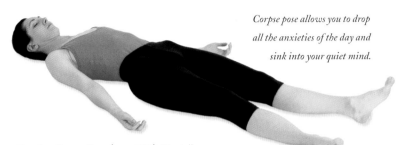

Corpse pose allows you to drop all the anxieties of the day and sink into your quiet mind.

Practice Corpse Pose (page 310). Mentally scan your body to become aware of any areas of tension or discomfort. Simply observe these areas—resist the urge to attach any judgment or emotionally loaded thought to them.

Next, move your attention slowly through your body from the top of your head down to your toes. Be with each part for a moment, then let that part relax. Accept each area of your body, however it feels.

When your whole body is relaxed, become aware of your feelings. Whatever you feel is just fine. Be with each feeling for a moment, then let it go. You are the passive observer of your feelings. Imagine a stream of fresh water washing it away. This pure, cleansing water flows through you. As this clear stream washes each feeling away, you will begin to experience feelings of peace and clarity inside.

After some time, become aware of any thoughts passing through your mind. Whatever you are thinking is just fine. Know that each thought will arise and then pass away. It is enough to be aware of each thought, like a silent witness, then let it go. Imagine a fresh breeze blowing through your mind, leaving it clear and empty.

Finally, allow yourself to rest in stillness. There is nothing to do or achieve. Simply be. You are not a human doing or acting, you are a human being. Let yourself exist in stillness. Just be.

Know that each time you practice this meditation, you will go deeper and receive more and more benefit.

To come out of this meditation, tune into your thoughts. Then move your awareness to your feelings once again. Deepen your awareness of your body as a single form, resting, relaxing. Let your body wake up, until you are ready to open your eyes. You will return restored, refreshed, and relaxed.

Guided Imagery—Visualization

Visualization is a powerful technique whereby you can become familiar with your imagination. The imagination is a wonderful tool that can be used to create particular states of mind and being. You can visualize colors, places, symbols, mandalas, gods, saints, or Tarot cards. People often choose an image that has a particular religious or spiritual meaning for them, or they choose something that they want to know more about. A good starting point is to find something of particular interest to you and focus on this same image over a number of meditation sessions. This allows your meditation to build momentum and can lead to stronger and more meaningful experiences. For the following meditation, you will imagine you are in nature. Keep the feeling light and playful until your imagination takes over and leads you deeper in. Allow fifteen minutes for this.

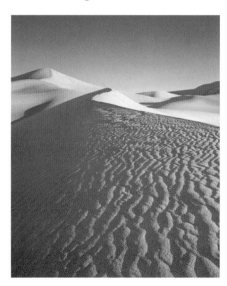

Visualization is based around an imagined image that is of interest to you.

- Sit or lie comfortably. Take some slow, deep, even breaths. Mentally sweep over your body to relax it part by part. Start with the crown of your head and work slowly down to your toes.

- Once you are relaxed, imagine yourself standing on a beach.

- See the beautiful, golden sand. You have a clear blue sky above you. Notice how the sunlight glints off the water. Observe how the branches of the trees sway in the gentle breeze.

- Hear the waves lapping on the shore, the gentle swish of the nearby trees, and the call of the seagulls flying overhead.

- Feel the sand between your toes, the sun warming your face and body, and the air caressing your skin.

- Smell and taste the fresh sea air.

- Become aware of the atmosphere or mood of

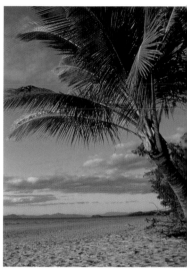

this place. What does it feel like actually to be here? Take some time to explore this place. You could go for a swim, or sunbathe, or walk down the beach.

- Return to the real world by becoming aware of your physical body. Take some long breaths so your body wakes up more with each inhalation. Listen to the sounds in the space around you. When you are ready, open your eyes.

Sound Meditation

Sound can be incorporated into your meditation through the use of a *mantra*—a word, phrase, or sentence that is repeated either aloud or internally. Using key words during meditation can have a very powerful effect because it focuses the mind and soothes the emotions.

Many Buddhists use the mantra *Om mane padme hum* (literally "the jewel is in the lotus"), while *Om nama shivaya*, a chant to the Hindu god Shiva, is popular in India. Mantras can be drawn from the Vedas (classic Indian texts), the Koran, the Bible, or any other scriptures. Many people find positive affirmations, such as "Every day in every way I am better, better, better," to be effective.

To practice a mantra meditation, sit or lie comfortably. Take some slow, deep breaths and let yourself fall into stillness. Bring to mind the mantra or affirmation of your choice and mentally repeat it in a rhythmic fashion. The nature of the mind is to wander, so whenever a thought, feeling, or sensation distracts you, gently bring your attention back to the sound of your mantra. When you notice your mind becoming more focused, let the mantra become softer and softer until you are resting in silence and stillness.

Chanting is another useful spiritual practice. Experiment with different sounds (such as sustained humming), words (such as the sacred syllable *Aum*) or any phrase that is meaningful to you. Using your own voice to make sustained vowel sounds, such as "aaaaaah," "eeeeeee," and "ooooooo," is called *toning*, and is especially powerful as a mental focusing and healing tool.

A mantra can be repeated rhythmically, either verbally or mentally.

The Present Moment—Five Senses Meditation

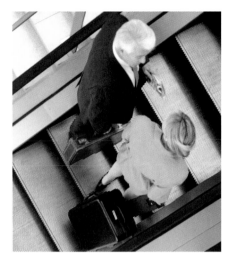

Practice mindfulness and sense awareness to help counteract everyday worries and concerns.

Being in the present moment is an extremely powerful experience. Aside from practicing the sensory awareness during meditation, integrating mindfulness and sense awareness into your everyday life will greatly improve your effectiveness and quality of life. Many find it a powerful tool to counter their habitual thoughts of worry and concern. Practice being continuously aware of a sense for as long as possible. For instance, become more mindful by acutely listening when someone else is speaking. Truly use your vision: What can you see as you walk or drive to work? Eat consciously by really tasting your food. Note its color, smell, and texture. Be aware of how your body feels before and after different foods. Enjoy some time in nature, being truly present. These practices lead you eventually to awaken into the fullness of the present moment.

This exercise lets you drop into the present moment by focusing on your physical senses. As you take ten or fifteen minutes for the Five Senses Meditation, you may also experience a delightful sense of stillness.

Sit or lie comfortably with your eyes closed. Let your breath deepen and become even and steady.

First, tune into the sense of smell. Become aware of what you can smell from moment to moment. Each time your mind wanders bring it back to this awareness.

● After two or three minutes, change your point of focus to observe the sense of taste. What do you taste on your tongue? Elsewhere in your mouth? Stay focused on this and simply observe.

● After several minutes, turn your attention to your vision. Open your eyes and see what you can see. Observe your sense of sight with perfect attentiveness.

● Close your eyes again. Be aware of touch. Can you feel the contact with your body against its supportive surface? Observe the touch of the cloth against your skin and the kiss of the air against your bare skin. Open yourself to the possibility of experiencing the sense of touch like never before.

● Next move to your sense of hearing. Listen to all the audible sounds from far away. Tune into the sounds in your immediate space. Tune into the sounds of your body. Listen acutely.

● Now turn inward and rest in the stillness. With nothing to do, allow yourself simply to be.

● Become aware of all your senses once again. Go through them one by one in reverse order: hearing, touch, sight, taste, and smell. Take some luxuriously slow, deep breaths. As you come out of this meditation, commit to observing your senses as you go about your tasks.

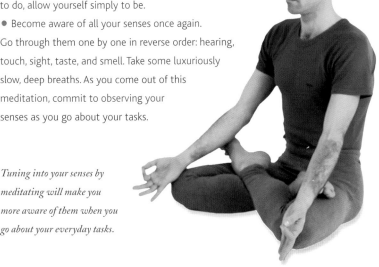

Tuning into your senses by meditating will make you more aware of them when you go about your everyday tasks.

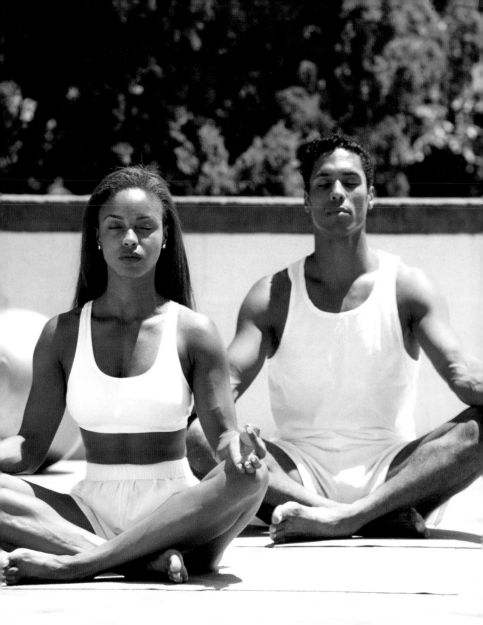

Finding
Your Yoga

Finding Your Yoga

The main form of yoga known in the West is Hatha yoga. Hatha yoga is an umbrella term that encompasses other commonly known physically based yogas, such as Iyengar yoga and Ashtanga Vinyasa yoga.

Less well known is a range of other yoga practices, which might be called branches of the tree of yoga. Let your yoga be flexible. Combine your practices in the way that best suits you. Read on to find your yoga.

Regardless of which branch or tradition of yoga appeals to you, a good teacher always helps. Do ask potential teachers about their qualifications. Keep in mind that the yoga industry is not as structured as law or accountancy. Although more and more teacher training programs are available, many very experienced and wonderful teachers don't hold a teaching certificate. What they do offer is a deep intuitive understanding, gleaned from years of disciplined practice. Another gauge is to ask potential teachers about their own personal practice. And, as with all of us, how they live their life will be a measure of how well they have integrated their yoga.

On the physical level, teachers will give valuable feedback on alignment and stimulate your mind with ways to stay present during the practice. However, remember that yoga is more than winding yourself up to resemble a pretzel—it's a whole philosophy, too. A yoga class might be a simple set of physical exercises or it might be spiced with life-enhancing ideas that arouse your interest, make you ponder, and encourage you to wonder at the mystery of life. Your journey into yoga is a personal one, so find a yoga tradition and a teacher with whom you feel a good connection. They might just turn out to be a helpful guide as you navigate your path through life.

Some types of yoga place an emphasis on mental, rather than physical, practices.

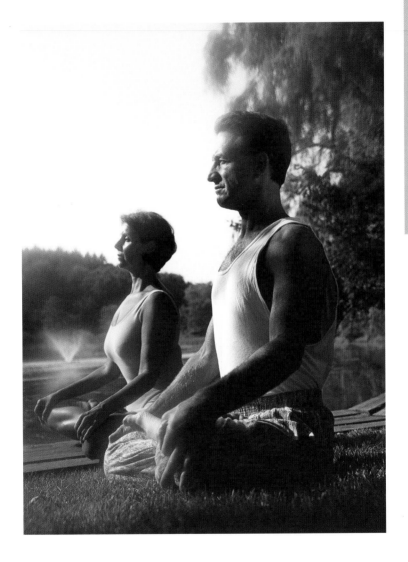

Nine Branches of the Tree of Yoga

While many people begin yoga to become more flexible or to cure their back pain, all the following paths of yoga aim for the same goal: the union of the individual consciousness with a universal consciousness. Each individual will have an affinity for one path over another—it depends on lifestyle, personality, and personal goals. The following are branches, some overlapping, from the tree of yoga. Feel free to blend them to create your own mix of integral yoga.

Bhakti Yoga

This is a devotional path with worship and service to God and/or a guru (a spiritual teacher). It often involves *kirtan* (chanting sessions). It cultivates a direct, intense relationship with the divine. Bhakti yoga suits those with an emotional and loving nature.

Hatha Yoga

Hatha yoga is philosophically rooted in the tantric movement. It uses the body as a tool for inner exploration. Hatha yoga aims to purify the body and therefore the mind. This is achieved through the use of *asana* (postures), *mudras* (gestures), *pranayama* (breath control) and *kriyas* (cleansing techniques).

Mentally repeating a mantra lies in the realm of Japa Yoga.

Hatha yoga uses movement to find the internal stillness.

The word *hatha*, composed of "sun" (*ha*) and "moon" (*tha*), conveys a feeling for a balance of complementary influences. Hatha yoga involves a combination of surrender and effort. The effort required explains why it is referred to as a yoga of force, where you reach union by direct effort, and also why Hatha yoga is ideal for those seeking good health and fitness.

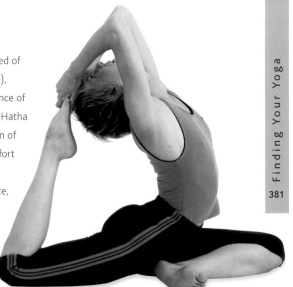

Japa Yoga (Mantra Yoga)

A mantra is a syllable, word, or phrase that can be repeated mentally, spoken aloud, or chanted. The use of a mantra aims to focus the mind and harmonize the body and may be intended in a devotional way, being toward God. Japa yoga is suitable for people who wish to withdraw from a noisy existence, those who are sensitive to sound vibrations and enjoy using their voice.

Jnana Yoga

Jnana yoga is also called the "yoga of true knowledge." Jnana yogics use self-study, reason and debate en route to wisdom. Jnana yoga suits those with rational, analytical minds who enjoy philosophy and are naturally introspective.

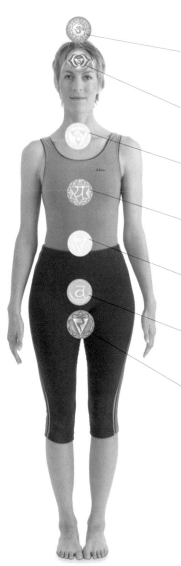

Crown center (*Sahasraha chakra*). This relates to spiritual illumination and the State of Bliss.

Brow center (*Anja chakra*). This relates to intuition and wisdom.

Throat center (*Visuddha chakra*). This relates to communication, self-expression, and truth.

Heart center (*Anahata chakra*). This relates to unconditional love, self-healing, and joy.

Solar plexus center (*Manifpura chakra*). This relates to power, will, and action.

Navel center (*Svadhisthana chakra*). This relates to creativity, sexuality, and relationships.

Base center (*Muladhara chakra*). This relates to stability, survival, and basic needs.

Laya yoga works with the seven energy centers (chakras) of the astral body, located from the base of the spine to the crown of the head. Chakras are "wheels of energy," the centers of force through which we receive, transmit, and process life energies.

Karma Yoga

This is the path of selfless service. The yoga is of action, where service is given without the expectation of reward. The action is dedicated to God, and the practitioner aims to let go of the fruits of the actions. Karma yogis believe that all actions (physical, verbal, mental) have consequences and we should be responsible for them. Karma yoga suits an active person who wishes to serve humanity.

Laya Yoga

This yoga involves special practices that work on the *chakras* (energy centers) to master the functions of each center. Also known as Kundalini yoga, this yoga can be very powerful, so it's best to seek out an experienced yoga teacher for guidance.

Raja Yoga

Known as the "kingly" path, Raja yoga develops control over the mind. Sometimes it is called classical yoga. Raja yoga uses will and meditation to improve the concentration, suspend the turnings of the mind, and achieve union.

Tantra Yoga

Tantra is rather misunderstood in the West because people often relate it to a type of spiritualized sex. In reality, sex is a very minor part of just one wing of Tantra. Tantra yoga uses renunciation, ritual, ceremonies, meditation, and mysticism. Hatha yoga is actually a branch of Tantra yoga.

Raja yoga uses self-inquiry via meditation.

Common Styles of Hatha Yoga

Hatha yoga is the umbrella term for yoga that uses physical practices to achieve the goals of yoga. Although any form of physical yoga is classified as Hatha yoga, if you attend a "Hatha yoga" class, it probably means a gentle form of yoga. While a Hatha yoga class is usually a general, slow-to-medium paced class, the style of teaching and level of difficulty varies from teacher to teacher—many Hatha yoga teachers have studied under various yoga traditions and combined them in their own personal way. Generally, a class will include posture work with emphasis on the breath, a final relaxation, and possibly little chanting or meditation. A Hatha yoga class is a good introduction to yoga and the postures are easily adapted to suit any level of student. The following are styles of Hatha yoga you may come across.

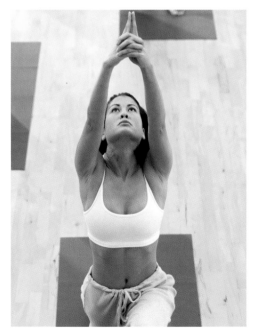

Hatha yoga is commonly practiced in the West. It concentrates primarily on posture and breath.

Ashtanga Vinyasa Yoga

If you want an aerobic workout, enjoy a good sweat, and want a toned, lean body, this could be the yoga for you. Ashtanga Vinyasa is a vigorous, dynamic form of yoga and it would benefit those seeking strength, flexibility, a clear mind, and an energy boost. This system of breath and connected movement combines Warming Breath (page 332) with a broad range of postures all linked together in a continuous flow—most postures are held for five breaths before moving on. It also uses the energy locks or *bandhas* (pages 338–41) and the eye gazing points (*drishti*, page 328) to focus the mind in a meditative way during the practice. With its emphasis on practice rather than theory, once a student learns the sequence, they are rather self-sufficient. K. Pattabhi Jois of Mysore in southern India helped make Ashtanga Vinyasa popular in the West and is recognized as the authority on it.

By practicing Ashtanga Vinyasa yoga, you get so warm that you'll notice an increase in your flexibility. As a set sequence, it is more difficult to adapt the postures to safeguard against any injuries you may have. In general, Ashtanga Vinyasa helps many people with back problems, but those with a tendency to knee problems need to take care. The demands of the poses combined with the tight hips of Westerners can put the knees at risk. Beginners need to start with a beginner's course or may prefer to start with a slower form of yoga.

Ashtanga Vinyasa yoga is vigorous and physically demanding.

Iyengar Yoga

Iyengar yoga takes a very precise view of the yoga postures. In an Iyengar yoga class, for example, you may hear the instructor talk about lifting the skin on the front of the armpits or be given detailed instructions on placement of the smallest toe. This attention to detail and deep understanding of the mechanics of the postures means it is an excellent place for beginners to start. It is well suited for those wanting to improve their posture or for those who have a specific health problem.

B.K.S. Iyengar was instrumental in bringing Iyengar yoga to the West in the 1960s, so many yoga teachers have practiced this form at one time or another along their path. Mr. Iyengar, who in his mid eighties, still teaches yoga in Pune, India. He believes the body has its own intelligence, and that by focusing on the body's physical alignment you can develop a full awareness and balance of your mind and body.

Unlike Ashtanga Vinyasa, where the breath is integral to the practice, Iyengar yoga brings focus on the breath at a much later stage, preferring to wait until a certain level of understanding of *asana* has been achieved. Iyengar yoga generally features long posture holding times. It makes use of props, such as blankets, foam pads, wooden blocks, and belts, to help achieve and maintain correct alignment. These props mean that this form of yoga is easily adapted to cater to different levels of strength, experience, and flexibility. Although a class may start with a short chant, you won't usually practice long meditations or breath work in an Iyengar class, and teachers usually zero in more on body mechanics than on aspects of the heart.

Iyengar yoga places great importance on precision of alignment.

Satyananda Yoga

Satyananda yoga takes a very holistic approach. Classes cover *asana*, *pranayama* and internal cleansing techniques alongside the more meditative practices of the Raja, Kundalini, Jnana, and Kriya yogas. Since all bases are covered, there is something to appeal to everyone, whether they are more devotionally, intellectually, or physically inclined.

Satyananda yoga encourages development of awareness of the self. Every class will offer a variety of postures, including limbering exercises aimed to build and streamline energy flow. Satyananda classes include *pranayama* (breath work), deep relaxation (yoga *nidra*), and meditation. Satyananda is very well suited to those attracted to the spiritual and philosophical aspects of yoga.

The very dedicated group of people who practice Satyananda yoga and convey a joyful energy are fortunate enough to have two living gurus. Swami Naranjan was trained from childhood to head up the school, while the founder, Swami Satyananda, has retired to live mainly in seclusion.

Swami Satyananda initiated many community projects, taking yoga classes to jails, schools, and hospitals. He was the first Indian guru to push for Westerners, particularly Western women, to be allowed to take their vows as *swamis* (Hindu monks). The school's northern Indian headquarters, the Bihar School of Yoga, is now a government-accredited yoga university that offers courses to degree level.

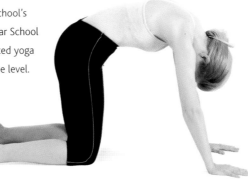

The emphasis of Satyananda yoga is spirituality and awareness of the self.

Kundalini Yoga

This is a spiritual school of yoga suited to those who are inclined toward meditation and who seek a higher state of consciousness. *Kundalini* is the name given to the energy that lies dormant at the base of the spine. This form of yoga seeks to awaken this energy (likened to a sleeping serpent) and to release the dormant power within each and every one of us as we get in touch with the core essence of who we are.

Kundalini yoga features many series of targeted practices. While a Kundalini class will vary from week to week, if you have a particular goal in mind, your teacher may recommend a series of practices to follow consistently at home for forty days, ninety days, or even longer.

While one series (called a *kriya*) may be aimed at stimulating the immune system, another set awakens the heart *chakra*, and a third prepares the practitioner for deep meditation. The exercises in each *kriya* are recommended in a certain order, for a set time and for a certain number of days. You may find yourself holding the same posture for three minutes and combining it with the *bandhas* and long, deep breathing, or else Bellows Breath, the "breath of fire." Meditation is very much a goal of Kundalini yoga, which often features *mudras*, *mantras*, or chanting. Chants may be short, *chakra*-related *bija mantras* (seed sounds) or longer devotional chants.

The guru of Kundalini yoga, Yogi Bhajan, is a Sikh from India. He lives and teaches in New Mexico. His aim in coming to the West was not to gather disciples but simply to spread the teachings of yoga and he has had some success, since there are now centers worldwide. While the teachers often wear turbans in the Sikh tradition, you don't have to be a Sikh to practice or teach Kundalini yoga.

Kundalini yoga often uses Bellows Breath during asana *practice.*

Viniyoga

The much revered, late Shri T. Krishnamacharya developed Viniyoga. Krishnamacharya was a well-known yoga master and the teacher of B.K.S. Iyengar and K. Pattabhi Jois in southern India. Over his life he used various approaches to yoga, and these are the ones that Iyengar and Jois took with them and refined into their systems. Toward the end of his life, he found a softer approach—Viniyoga—and it is this that his son, T.K.V. Desikachar, has continued to the present day. Desikachar and his son Kausthub still leave their base in India, from which they teach and lecture about Viniyoga around the world.

Viniyoga is usually taught on a one-to-one basis and as such has great therapeutic capacity. In a Viniyoga lesson, your teacher will assess your current state (physically, mentally, and emotionally) and devise a yoga practice for you to continue at home. As a completely personal consultation it is truly holistic and well suited as a rebalancing practice for any sphere. It is ideal if you have special circumstances or a specific personal goal in mind. Your prescription may be based on any number of things: devotional or physical practices; chanting of the Vedas (texts of ancient knowledge); or breath work or meditation—things considered by some to be outside the realm of yoga might even be recommended, such as playing a musical instrument.

Viniyoga postures are often flowed into and then out of, in time with breathing.

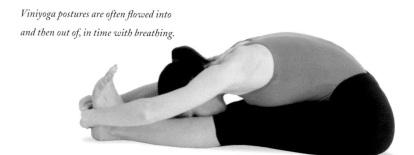

Bikram Yoga

The flamboyant, Los Angeles-based Bikram Choudury created this system of "Hot Yoga," which is geared toward people who don't mind the heat or beads of sweat dripping onto their mats. Bikram yoga is a standardized series of two breathing exercises and twenty-four poses followed by a relaxation, all aimed at addressing common health complaints and designed to be accessible to beginners.

Like Ashtanga Vinyasa yoga, each pose prepares the body for the one that follows. No props (besides the possibility of the wall) are used and no inverted postures are taught. There is also little in the way of upper body strengtheners.

The room, heated to temperatures of 90°–104°F (about 36–42°C), helps students sweat out toxins and stretch further than they ever have ever stretched before. While many rave about this new take on yoga and find the sequence invigorating, yoga in sauna-like conditions is not for everyone. While many students report feeling energized, a number of students feel faint after some time in the sweatbox. Bikram yoga, whose schools are called the Yoga College of India, is more for those ready to do battle with adversity than for those seeking the contemplation of a quietly meditative class.

As a set sequence, Bikram yoga may be less acceptable to those with particular health complaints.

Sivananda Yoga

This form of yoga is ideal for those who enjoy a mix of physical and devotional practices. Each class includes a little chanting plus some breathing exercises. Following this, *asanas* are practiced. Each yoga class includes the same twelve postures, which are designed to stimulate the *chakras*. Each *chakra* is stimulated as the emphasis of the postures moves progressively up from the base *chakra* (via a standing posture) to the crown *chakra* (via Headstand, which is not always suitable for beginners). A systematic final relaxation is practiced in each class.

Sivananda yoga is good for beginners because it allows them to get used to the same sequence and have the chance to deepen their understanding of the postures it involves. For the same reason, it might not be the tradition of choice for those who prefer more variety to their practice. Sivananda places less emphasis on alignment and more emphasis on chanting and breathwork than many of the other Hatha yoga schools.

The Sivananda group was founded by the late Swami Vishnu Devananda, who was a disciple of Swami Sivananda (Swami Sivananda was also the guru of Swami Satyananda). Now run by a group of mostly Western *swamis*, they have centers and ashrams around the world run by seekers in various stages of renunciation, who strongly embrace the spiritual aspects of yoga.

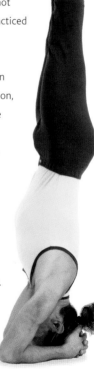

As each Sivananda yoga class features the same postures, beginners can pace themselves.

Glossary

Adho Downward.

Anguli Toes.

Anjana Name of the mother of Hanuman, a powerful Hindu monkey chief.

Ardha Half.

Asana Posture or pose.

Baddha Bound.

Bandha An energy lock or seal in the body.

Bharadva The name of a sage.

Bheka Frog.

Bodymind All aspects of the individual—physical, psychological, emotional, and spiritual.

Chandra Moon.

Danda Staff or rod.

Dhanura Bow.

Dharana Concentration.

Dhyana Meditation.

Dristhi Gaze.

Dvi Two or both.

Eka One.

Gheranda A sage, the author of the *Gheranda Samitha*.

Go Cow.

Hala Plough.

Hasta Hand.

Hatha The yoga of effort.

Jala Water.

Jalan A net or network.

Janu Knee.

Jathara Abdomen

Kapota Pigeon or dove.

Karani Active.

Kasyapa A legendary sage, father of the gods and of the demons.

Kriya A cleansing process.

Kundalini An energy, likened to the snake that is said to lie coiled at the base of the spine.

Kurma Tortoise.

Maha Great, mighty, noble.

Mala A garland or wreath.

Mantra A hymn or word, repeated.

Marichi A sage, son of Brahma.

Matsya Fish.

Mayura Peacock.

Mudra A position that creates an energy seal in the body.

Mukha Mouth or face.

Mula Root.

Nadis Energy channels in the body.

Neti Nose cleansing.

Nidra Sleep.

Nirlamba Unsupported.

Pada Leg or foot.

Padma Lotus.

Parigha A beam or bar used to close a gate.

Parivrtta Turned around, revolved.

Parsva Side, lateral.

Paschima The West.

Patanjali Yoga philosophizer. Author of the *Yoga-sutras*.

Pinda Fetus, embryo.

Prana Breath, respiration, life, vitality, wind, energy, strength. It also connotes the soul.

Pranayama Rhythmic control of the breath. The fourth stage of yoga and the hub around which the wheel of yoga revolves.

Prasarita Spread out, stretched out.

Raja Lord or king.

Salamba Supported.

Sama Same, equal, or even.

Samadhi The eighth and highest stage of yoga. A state in which there is a feeling of supreme joy and peace.

Sarvanga The whole body.

Sasanka Hare, rabbit.

Sava A corpse.

Setu bandha Bridge construction.

Sirsa Head.

Sodhana Purification, cleansing.

Sukha Happiness, delight, joy, pleasure, comfort.

Supta Reclined.

Tada Mountain.

Tan To stretch, extend, lengthen out.

Tittibha Firefly.

Trataka To look or to gaze.

Tri Three.

Ud To fly.

Upavista Seated.

Urdhva Raised, elevated, upward.

Ustra Camel.

Ut Intense.

Utthita Extended.

Vasistha A legendary sage.

Viloma Against the order of things.

Viparita Inversion, inverted, reversed.

Virahadra Name of a great warrior.

Vritti Mode of being, condition.

Vrksa Tree.

Yana Upward.

Yoga This word is derived from the root *Yuj* meaning to join, to yoke, to concentrate attention on. It is one of the six systems of Indian philosophy collated by the sage Patanjali. The chief aim of yoga is to teach the means by which the human soul may be completely united with the Supreme Spirit.

Yoga-sutras The classical work on yoga by the Indian sage, Patanjali.

Index

Acknowledgments

Dedication

Developing the ability to be in the present moment is a reward in itself.
To me, yoga practice is about re-remembering who I am. Another instant reward
comes from my students when I see the flicker of recognition cross their faces
during a class and I realize they just "got" it too. For this I thank them.

I have been blessed with many wonderful teachers around the world.
My special thanks go to these people for their help in the more recent past.

Simon Borg Olivier, a walking example of a high *prana* state, who inspires me
with his knowledge, mastery, creativity, and love of all things *asana*.

Julie Henderson's mix of body centering and Buddhism flicked the switch in me
that unfolded the deep comprehension of the feeling of internal spaciousness.

Thanks to Stephen Cottee for reminding me to
"remember to remember." In teaching me about the
nature of recentering, his meditations have been
enormously life enhancing.

And thanks to Michael Popplewell for his
friendship over the whole of my adult life.
He applies his special combination of "real
life" practicality with profound spiritual
wisdom in a way that few can match.

Bridgewater Books would like to thank the following for the permission to
reproduce copyright material: Corbis pp. 11/12,16, 22, 29, 376.